A Parent Guide to Strabismus, Eye Muscle Surgery & Vision Therapy

Steve Gallop, OD

Optometric Extension Program Foundation

Published by Optometric Extension Program Foundation, Inc.
1921 East Carnegie Ave., 3-L
Santa Ana, CA 92705-5811
Managing Editor: Sally Marshall Corngold

Library of Congress Cataloging-in-Publication Data

Gallop, Steve.
    A parent guide to strabismus, eye muscle surgery & vision therapy / Steve Gallop, OD.
        pages cm
    ISBN 978-0-929780-40-5 (alk. paper)
    1. Strabismus--Surgery--Popular works. 2. Strabismus--Treatment--Popular works. 3. Pediatric ophthalmology--Popular works. I. Optometric Extension Program Foundation. II. Title.
    RE771.G35 2014
    618.92'0977--dc23
                                                2014026634

****

Optometry is the health care profession specifically licensed by state law to prescribe lenses, optical devices and procedures to improve human vision. Optometry has advanced vision therapy as a unique treatment modality for the development and remediation of the visual process. Effective vision therapy requires extensive understanding of:

- the effects of lenses (including prisms, filters and occluders)

- the variety of responses to the changes produced by lenses

- the various physiological aspects of the visual process

- the pervasive nature of the visual process in human behavior

    As a consequence, effective vision therapy requires the supervision, direction and active involvement of the optometrist.

****

TABLE OF CONTENTS

DEDICATION

This book is dedicated to all the people who honor me with the opportunity to help them have more comfortable, effective visual process and hopefully a better life.

ACKNOWLEDGMENTS

The author wishes to acknowledge his favorite mother and proof reader Jeanie Gallop, who despite the most extenuating of circumstances, managed to find fault with her oldest son (at his request for a change). I wouldn't be where I am today (or anywhere for that matter) without her and I'd surely have many more typos. Responsibility for any remaining errors lies at the feet of the author and no one elf else.

THANKS

Thanks to the Optometric Extension Program Foundation (OEPF) for its many decades of service to the profession of optometry, especially those who practice with a behavioral/developmental philosophy. Thanks, also, for almost three decades of supporting and enhancing my professional development, which has which has enabled me to continue improving my ability to provide care for those who seek my help.

Thanks, also, to Dr. Paul Harris, cuerrent president of OEPF, for finding value in the information I present here, and to Sally Corngold for help in the preparation of this manuscript for publication.

Introduction

Do you know someone whose eyes look kind of funny? When you look at them, does it seem that one of their eyes is looking at you as the other eye gazes at their nose or at some unknown object off to the side? Do you get an uncomfortable sensation when you speak to them face to face, uncertain of how to look at them? Many people have difficulty using their eyes as a team. Sometimes it appears obvious, sometimes not. Most of us have had the experience of seeing someone who has an eye that doesn't seem to be aiming where it should. If this is confusing or uncomfortable for us, imagine what it might be like for them.

Do you have a child with and eye that seems to be pointing in the wrong direction or do yourself have an eye that wanders? Are you self-conscious when other people look at you? Do you worry that they keep thinking about which eye they should look at and where your other eye is looking? Do you get frustrated when you look in the mirror and see that one eye is not cooperating? Have you considered having surgery to straighten that eye? Are you worried that surgery is dangerous? Do you wonder if it really works or if there is some better alternative? There is usually more than one way to solve a problem, and improving the alignment and function of two eyes that don't seem to be coordinating with each other is that type of problem.

Although we have two eyes, they need to work as a single, integrated unit. They must move, aim, and focus in unison at all times in order for the visual process to function as it was meant to function. There are many levels of eye teaming difficulty, from the very mild, where the eyes look normal and straight, to the more significant degree described above, where it is obvious to any casual observer that they two eyes are not looking at the same thing at the same time.

Can you and your children enjoy 3-D movies? Are they really in 3-D for you and for them? People with eye teaming problems like strabismus are not likely to see in 3-D as we are meant to do. Some can see in 3-D, but it is an effort and they walk out of the movie feeling odd or even nauseated. We need our two eyes to work with a considerable amount of integration and stamina, and a minimum of effort in order to see in 3-D on a consistent basis, especially for 3-D movies. We have two eyes facing forward because we are meant to see in 3-D. Each eye sees a slightly different view of the world; the brain combines these two views of the world into an integrated whole, which, when things are working as they are supposed to, provides us with a 3-D view of the world. Many people with significant eye teaming problems, like strabismus, do not actually see the world in 3-D, though they may have no awareness that this is the case. Chapter 4 introduces vision therapy, which is the best way to help someone learn how to see in 3-D if that is not happening automatically for them. Most people with strabismus can improve their eye teaming and the ability to see in 3-D with vision therapy.

These problems can and often do remain undetected, or at least not properly addressed, for a person's whole life when there is no cosmetic aspect to make the eye teaming difficulty obvious.

The more severe cases of eye teaming problems are easily noticed by others. We all know or have seen someone who has one eye that appears to turn in a different direction from the fellow eye. These problems can and often do remain undetected, or at least not properly addressed, for a person's whole life when there is no cosmetic aspect to the eye teaming difficulty. A person may have various complaints regarding comfort and/or efficiency in these cases. It is entirely possible that these people would be surprised to learn that there was some problem with their vision because they can often see clearly, either with or without glasses or contact lenses, and because they have never been exposed to any way of seeing other than what they have known throughout their lives. They have not been given any options to explore because most eye care professionals have intentionally decided to ignore these kinds of issues, and therefore are likely to miss the opportunity to assist these people in achieving a higher level of visual performance and greater visual comfort. The main reason for this is that most eye doctors are comfortable with the idea that their main task is for people to see clearly—nothing else really matters, except that the eyes themselves are free of disease or damage. Don't get me wrong, healthy eyes are important and clear eyesight is generally a good thing, but there is much more to optimal visual performance. Less than optimal visual performance can often be a significant obstacle to reaching our potential.

People with subtle eye teaming issues may have any number of complaints that they don't realize are related to how their visual system is working. This includes complaints such as double vision, trouble reading, poor handwriting, headaches, eye fatigue, dry eyes, motion sickness and poor coordination. These complaints will never be attributed to the actual causes, which are often eye teaming and/or focusing problems, without a proper evaluation by a *behavioral optometrist*. The vast majority of people fitting this description can achieve excellent improvement in performance and comfort by working with a behavioral optometrist who offers vision therapy and therapeutic lenses as treatment.

Many people are unaware that their vision is not working properly, since they have nothing to which they can compare it. They may simply avoid activities that cause discomfort, frustration, or fatigue, or they may not realize that the symptoms they experience are visually related. Still others have long-term, constant, nagging problems that are frequently written off by their doctors as insignificant, imaginary, or totally unrelated to their eyes. People in this category are also very likely to benefit from what behavioral optometry has to offer.

The following pages will, for the most part, be dedicated to the more severe cases. That is, those whose general cosmetic appearance has been affected by the eyes' extreme inability to work properly as a team, causing them to consider eye muscle surgery as a resolution.

It is those who have cosmetically noticeable eye turns who are most likely to wind up consulting a surgeon. Surgeons are unlikely to consider alternative possibilities for straightening the eyes, especially since many are convinced that surgery is the only known treatment for the condition. Unfortunately, even in the 21st century, the most well-known and probably most common primary intervention for a turned eye remains eye muscle surgery. These surgeries are touted as cures for cosmetically misaligned eyes, but unlike most other cosmetic surgeries, eye muscle surgery is covered by medical insurance. I believe this is because there is a pretense that by making the eyes look straight they will automatically work together. Unfortunately, nothing could be further from the truth. The ability of the two eyes to work as a cohesive unit is just one complex aspect of an even more intricate visual process, as will be shown throughout this book.

These eye muscle surgeries rarely, and then mostly by chance, result in a properly functioning visual system. Some surgeons even claim that eye muscle surgery can also cure *amblyopia*, commonly known as *lazy eye.* Although the term lazy eye can also be used to describe an eye that does not look straight, it is usually meant to refer to an eye that cannot see 20/20 - usually much worse. Amblyopia is a condition where one eye cannot see as well as the other eye no matter what lens is tried.

Behavioral optometrists expect the visual system to perform at a high level throughout our lives.

A properly functioning visual system is one that includes consistent high-level eye teaming with excellent depth perception. The visual system is meant to continue operating at a high level indefinitely. Unfortunately, eye muscle surgeries are routinely sold to the public as the only way to fix the problem. These pronouncements are often accompanied by warnings that not submitting to the procedure could result in blindness in the affected eye. A number of parents have told me that they were warned of this by surgeons. In addition, it is common for surgeons to present other types of intervention as experimental, ineffective, and/or dangerous quackery.

Every year thousands of children and adults are diagnosed with conditions known as crossed eyes, wall eyes, or lazy eyes. The technical term is *strabismus,* when the two eyes are obviously not pointing at the same place at the same time. Esotropia is when one or both eyes appear to cross improperly, exotropia is when one or both eyes tend to turn away from each other inappropriately. There is also vertical strabismus, where one eye aims higher than the other, though this is less common and rarely severe enough to present a cosmetic problem - the most famous exception being Abraham Lincoln; in fact, the sculptor of the Lincoln Memorial was so keen on detail and accuracy that you can see this in the statue.

Cosmetically noticeable eye turns are frequently treated by surgical means. One or more eye muscles may be repositioned to alter the cosmetic alignment of the eyes. Some surgeons prefer to operate on the problematic eye, some on the other eye; some will operate on both eyes. There are numerous techniques and procedures available. While the quality and safety of these procedures has improved over the years, there has been little change in the philosophy of most surgeons who are diagnosing and treating these conditions, and therefore little change in the quality of the outcomes.

This surgery-based philosophy presumably maintains that there is some problem with the eye muscles when the two eyes are not aiming properly. While eye muscle damage can actually happen, it is quite rare. Many people experience less than satisfactory results after surgery because of the limitations of this philosophy. Problems may surface immediately following the operation or may take several years to become noticeable. At this point, I am referring to eye alignment problems. There is absolutely no guarantee that eyes which appear straight immediately after surgery will stay that way.

Actually, the need for multiple operations is quite common. Many people have unsatisfactory results from eye muscle surgery because the eyes are merely part of an intricate visual process that mostly occurs in the brain.

When a surgically straightened eye deviates again, surgeons simply see this as an indication of the need for further surgery. Actually, the need for multiple operations is quite common when the standard medical/surgical approach is taken. Unfortunately, because of differing philosophies, all of these people must continue with their vision as it is, or attempt further surgery, unless they are fortunate enough to find a doctor who understands their problems from a different perspective. They need a doctor who knows how to work with them to achieve improvement through non-surgical means—a behavioral optometrist. This book addresses all these issues, as well as presenting alternatives for treating these conditions before surgery, instead of with surgery or after surgery.

One problem that arises initially, in most cases, is that parents and patients seeking guidance and help are given limited information. People generally seek a specialist when a vision problem is significant enough to cause concern. This is particularly true when the problem is cosmetically apparent. Such cases include eyes that turn in or out, and/or a significant difference between the two eyes' ability to see clearly. Most people seek expert advice in such cases and often end up in the office of an ophthalmologist. An ophthalmologist is a medical doctor, a specialist highly trained in diagnosing and treating all eye diseases, typically using medications and other invasive measures such as surgery. The other branch of eye care professionals are optometrists. An optometrist is a doctor trained in diagnosing and treating a variety of eye health problems. Optometrists are permitted to use medications to treat certain common conditions.

Optometrists and ophthalmologists are licensed to prescribe lenses and treat functional and developmental vision problems like strabismus and amblyopia. In fact, the lines of distinction are becoming increasingly blurred as optometrists continually expand their scope of practice in the direction of ophthalmology. An important distinction must be made in choosing a professional to evaluate, diagnose, and provide treatment options when dealing with the types of functional and developmental vision problems that are so often treated with eye muscle surgery.

Anyone considering eye muscle surgery for themselves or their child should consult a Behavioral Optometrist to get a broader understanding of how the visual process works and how surgery fits into the bigger picture. Many eye teaming problems can be corrected, or greatly reduced, through non-surgical means.

There is a specialty area within optometry known as Behavioral or Developmental Optometry. Behavioral optometrists specialize in diagnosing and treating functional and developmental conditions of the visual system. These doctors will treat such visual problems without the use of surgery and in most cases without drugs. In those cases where surgery is unavoidable for one reason or another, these doctors will work with the patient before and after surgery to optimize the outcome whenever possible.

The conditions at issue here are known as binocular vision problems, that is, problems with the way the eyes work as a team. I am mainly going to address the various types of strabismus and amblyopia. It is rare that both eyes are amblyopic, but this can occur. Cases requiring surgery make up a minority of such vision problems, and developmental/behavioral optometrists believe that non-surgical options should be investigated before deciding on the need for surgery. Many eye teaming problems can be corrected or greatly reduced through non-surgical means (lenses, prisms, and vision therapy), which will be discussed later. Because of these other safer and less invasive options, surgery should be a last resort in most cases, although many who are considered experts, in particular ophthalmologists, feel that it is a first choice, or the only choice. In fact, eye muscle surgery is the second most common eye surgery performed.[1,2]

The visual process is not an eye process, but more a brain process. The visual process is pervasive in human behavior and development.

Vision is a complicated process that is not fully understood by most of the public. In fact, even though vision is the most studied and well understood of all our senses, science still does not fully understand the entire process of vision. One thing we do know is that the visual process is not an eye process; it is a brain and body process. The visual process is pervasive in human behavior and development. The eyes themselves are fairly complex structures, but their main purpose is to absorb light and convert that light into chemical signals, which then become electrical signals that travel to and from many parts of the brain and body. It is important to think in terms of seeing with our brains rather than with our eyes. It is also important to understand that the primary purpose of the visual process is to *direct action*.

The visual process develops throughout our lives. The visual process is learned and therefore is trainable at any age.

Before we go any further, I would like to explain my working definition of the term *vision*. Actually, I will generally avoid the term vision. I will replace it with *visual process* since most people, including most eye care professionals, already have their own definition of the word vision and consider it to be nothing more than the ability to see clearly - I call this eyesight. The visual process is much more than that. It is a dynamic process that occurs in the brain. The visual process develops, and it continues to do so throughout our lives. The visual process is learned and therefore is trainable at any age.

The visual process is about deriving meaning and *directing action* in response to light entering the eyes. Reading a series of letters on a wall chart or even using more modern devices is nothing more than a measurement of eyesight or visual acuity, which is only one of many important aspects of the visual process; in many cases, it is not even the most important aspect. The visual process is tied in to the way we see the world, the way we think about the world, and the options that seem available to us as we go through life. It is intimately related to our overall development and our performance in school, work, sports, and recreation. We are more dependent on the visual process as a means of interacting with our environment than with any of our other senses. As optometrists utilizing a behavioral philosophy of the visual process have understood for almost 100 years, the visual process is an important aspect of all human behavior.

Our two eyes must function as a single unit to provide comfortable, effective input. Consistently reliable input is necessary for optimal information processing and meaningful, accurate responses. The ability of the eyes to coordinate with each other (binocular vision, stereo vision or eye teaming) is what allows us to perceive things as being three dimensional, and to understand and make sense of the space that surrounds us, as well as the people and things with whom we share that space at any given time. For example, if the eyes are not coordinating properly, a person may experience double vision. As you can imagine, this is very disruptive and troubling to deal with.

Poor eye teaming often leads to errors in judging distances and depth (space) whether or not there is double vision. This in turn affects the way we move through a room, play with toys or other people, color within the lines, and perform every activity that requires us to move any part of our body with some purpose in mind. This is especially important for driving a car. If we cannot accurately judge space, our reactions to traffic or parking situations will be less than optimal. The accuracy of eye teaming is critical in reading, writing, and learning in general. Good eye teaming is also important for athletic performance.

Poor eye teaming can cause people to feel insecure in social situations. People with noticeable eye turns are often self-conscious. People feel awkward around them because it can be strange to look someone in the eye while watching the other eye look elsewhere. People with eye teaming problems often find it difficult to make or maintain eye contact even with family members. Therefore, the visual process is often a critical aspect of human social behavior and development.

Many people considered candidates for eye muscle surgery have managed to overcome their visual problems non-surgically, or have found higher level improvement by adding vision therapy to other treatments.

Over the years, behavioral optometrists have worked with millions people of all ages, with all types of functional vision problems. Our experiences in working with people in this way have shown that there is almost always potential for meaningful improvement in visual function and development. This includes children with various learning problems, people with eye turns, lazy eyes, and those who have suffered brain injuries or are living with various developmental and/or neurological deficits. Many of these people would be considered candidates for eye muscle surgery but have managed to overcome their visual problems non-surgically, or have found higher level improvement by adding vision therapy to other treatments.

Behavioral optometrists also have the good fortune to be able to help those who have had eye muscle surgeries that did not turn out as hoped. These people suffer on a daily basis because of the inability of their eyes to work together, and they seek specialized care to make them more comfortable. The main goal of this book is to provide more comprehensive information about the available options than what is typically offered. It is also my goal to provide an overview of the factors affecting visual function, an understanding of the ways good visual performance and comfort can be achieved, and the stories of some people who have had experience in all these areas.

Chapter One

THE VISUAL PROCESS

Vision means very different things to different people. Most eye care professionals consider vision to be the ability to make out a certain size letter at a certain distance; this is typically tested with the patient sitting in a chair looking at several rows of letters on the wall or by having the person look into a device capable of taking and recording this measurement. The more modern device is considerably less reliable than the old fashioned eye chart, as it turns out. Also, as an aside, the interested practitioner can get a great deal of information about the person while observing them as they read the eye chart. I prefer not to leave this task either to technicians or mechanical devices for that very reason. Most eye care providers view this ability to see clearly as an eyeball phenomenon, and call it vision. I prefer to label it eyesight.

Behavioral optometrists have, over many decades, developed a much more in-depth impression of vision, which is based on our experiences and our understanding of the visual process. Either way, the ability to see clearly with or without lenses is merely a part of a complex and dynamic visual process. We have learned that the visual process is the result of a "simple" eye and a complex brain. While it is not entirely fair to describe the human eye as simple, it is relatively simple in contrast to the amazing complexity of the visual process as a whole. The visual process is pervasive in human behavior. By that I mean that the visual process has an important role in just about everything we do. It helps us manage our relationship to gravity, helping us to remain upright and to balance as we move. It helps us follow a line of print for reading and guides our hand across the page as we write.

The visual process is a dynamic process of taking in information, processing that information in order to attach some meaning to it, and most importantly, planning and executing some response to the information.[3] A response may be in the form of thought, physical action, or both. This means that the visual process is not merely a way of passively acquiring information. It is a dynamic process that sends and receives information from throughout the brain and body. The visual process is also a fundamental aspect of formulating and carrying out responses to the incoming information. I will therefore be using the phrase *visual process* to refer to what is really at issue whenever we consider evaluating and treating any challenges that involve what we see and how we act.

Most life on our planet is dependent upon sunlight. We need light for many aspects of health and survival, which is not surprising since we inhabit a *solar* system. Vision, or more accurately, a light-sensing apparatus, first evolved as a means of orienting tiny creatures to the light and to their broader environment. This provided them with information about their own orientation in relation to their environment. The visual process in humans is still involved with this same fundamental issue. There are other issues that have been added on, but the basic element of orienting ourselves within our three-dimensional environment and in relation to gravity remains important.

The visual process is about obtaining meaning and directing action as a result of light entering the eyes. As light enters the eyes through the pupils, it passes through the interior of the eyes and across the back of the eyes - the retinas. This distribution of light provides information about the lighted environment and our place within it. The lighted environment is a volume of space, inhabited by people, animals, and things with which we must relate and interact. Once the light enters our eyes, we must process whatever meaning there may be for us, and then we must formulate and carry out some type of response, which could include doing absolutely nothing.

The visual process is concerned with several basic components that deal with several fundamental concepts:

- **Our own orientation within the environment,**
- **Our understanding of the space between us and other things in the environment,**

- **Our ability accurately to recognize the various components of the environment,**

- **Our ability to interact with the whole of our moment-to-moment environment as well as to utilize previous information and images,**

- **Our ability to anticipate and plan for what is coming next, and**

- **Our ability to communicate internally and to others about our visual experiences.**

The visual process is initially concerned with understanding our relationship to gravity. This tells us about our posture and our orientation, how we are and where we are. The visual process interacts with the vestibular system to help us know when we are in motion or stationary. Motion sickness, dizziness, and other movement, orientation and balance challenges often respond to vision therapy when the visual system is at the root of the problem, which is very common. We must also have a reasonably accurate understanding of the nature and purpose of the other components of our immediate environment. This provides better context about our position within our surroundings and how we might want or need to interact with it. Our ability to process the nature of the physical environment and our own postural status is the basis for our ability to initiate and successfully carry out movement.

The visual process also enables us to appreciate and understand our interrelationship with the other aspects of our environment. It informs us as to where these other things are in relation to us. Once we are able to determine where things are, we can know where to direct our attention to further investigate these aspects of the environment, so we might know exactly what they are and what they mean to us. All of this is hopefully happening not in sequence, but simultaneously and without any conscious effort on our part. All this information enables us to formulate thoughts, feelings, learning, decision making, problem solving, and communication with others. The effort involved may not be conscious, but it is considerably greater when there are disturbances in the visual process, such as poor eye teaming.

Optimally, the visual process will continue to develop as long as we continue using it, since the demands we face change throughout our lives.

Visual development is another important aspect of the picture we are trying to paint here. The visual process begins to develop within the womb and must continue to develop after we are born and throughout our lives. Optimally, the visual process will continue to develop, to some degree, as long as we continue using it, since the demands we face change throughout our lives. Just as we cannot walk when we are born, we cannot use our visual process to its fullest at this time. Even with healthy legs, we must go through developmental stages of creeping and crawling prior to walking upright. This is in part due to muscle development, but is mostly due to neurological development, including an appropriate level of sophistication of the visual process.

Developmentally speaking, we begin by emphasizing our mouths and then our hands to explore objects around us, then combining the eyes and hands in increasingly complex ways, and finally achieving the ability to interact with objects visually without the need to physically touch them. One reason some children seem to grab everything they can get their hands on is that they are still under-utilizing the visual process. They are essentially still using their sense of touch to "see." Behavioral optometrists use terms like reach, grasp, and release when evaluating and describing the interactions of the visual process with various aspects of the environment. The concept of visual development is usually neglected by general eye care practitioners, but is a cornerstone of the thinking and practice of behavioral optometrists. Understanding the importance of visual development helps us appreciate that the visual process can be at various levels of proficiency and can be modified in some way.

Visual performance may be at different levels during different activities, and as a result of differing physical, emotional, or stress levels. The visual process can be and in fact is modified by the individual on an ongoing basis. This typically occurs on a subconscious level, without the benefit of professional guidance that is based on sound philosophy and clinical experience. For example, if an infant or young child has an eye that drifts out of alignment with the other eye, the brain accesses the various aspects of the visual process to find the most effective way to carry out daily tasks under those conditions. Sometimes attempts to keep the two eyes working as a cohesive unit are successful, or at least relatively so, and sometimes the attempts are unsuccessful. One response to such a visual difficulty is to keep the uncooperative eye turned so far out of alignment that the brain can, for all intents and purposes, ignore that eye (to avoid seeing double) and carry on with life fairly well. This of course introduces another problem, the cosmetic issue.

Vision therapy is a process by which problems in any area(s) of visual development and function can be prevented, reduced, or eliminated in a completely safe, noninvasive manner.

Visual performance can also be modified with the help of a knowledgeable practitioner who has some understanding of the factors and possibilities involved. This is likely to result in a much better and longer lasting positive outcome. This brings us to the concept of *visual training* or *vision therapy*, which will be discussed in more depth later. Briefly, vision therapy is a process by which problems in any area(s) of visual development and function can be prevented, reduced, or eliminated in a completely safe, noninvasive manner. It involves the active participation of the individual in their own healing process and is almost completely without risk of unwanted side effects when properly performed.

The standard approach to eye care subscribed to by almost all MDs and the majority of optometrists (ODs) on the one hand and the developmental/ functional/behavioral approach to vision care practiced by behavioral optometrists lead to very different styles of evaluating and treating all types of visual problems. The approach to near- and farsightedness, astigmatism, so-called lazy eye, eye turns, etc., will be very different depending on the background and philosophy of the practitioner. The medical approach treats vision as an eyeball phenomenon, and doctors who practice this way will typically be satisfied knowing that the eyes are free of physical disease or damage and can see the 20/20 line on the chart, with or without lenses. While these issues are certainly important, other issues, especially those of a functional or developmental nature, tend to go unrecognized because they lie outside the context of the typical eye exam.

There are several areas of visual performance that are essential to evaluate: eye movements, eye teaming, focusing, peripheral visual awareness, and visual acuity.

Those subscribing to the developmental/functional/behavioral philosophy see vision as a dynamic process that involves the eyes, the brain, and the body. They will need to evaluate the visual process in much greater depth to feel they have an understanding of the person's visual process, developmental status, behavior, and needs. Behavioral optometrists are interested not only in clear eyesight and healthy eyes, but also in understanding how an individual uses the enormous potential of the visual process to meet their daily needs. We are interested in understanding the role of the visual process in human behavior and how we can improve a person's life through the optimal utilization of the visual process.

There are several areas of visual performance that are essential to evaluate. These are eye movements, eye teaming, focusing, peripheral visual awareness, and visual acuity, all with an eye toward understanding a person's current level of visual development and the potential for future improvement.

Eye movements have three main categories that are pertinent to our discussion: pursuits, fixations, and saccades. Pursuit eye movements are used to track a moving target, like watching a bird in flight. Fixation is the ability to look directly and steadily at a specific object for a meaningful period of time, which can vary depending on the requirements of the particular circumstances. Saccades are used to switch fixation rapidly and accurately from one object to another. The main point is that the eyes should be under the control of the individual and not the other way around. We should be able to move our eyes when we so choose and we should be able to look at something for as long as we like, all without giving it a second thought and without any discomfort whatsoever.

We should be able to move our eyes without the need to move our head or other parts of our bodies in many circumstances. These skills permit easy shifting of the eyes along the line of print in a book, a rapid and accurate return to the next line, and quick, accurate shifts between desk and chalkboard. You can imagine many more examples in everyday life. Fixation ability is closely related to the ability to maintain visual and mental attention. Inability to maintain fixation will adversely affect the ability to mentally attend for appropriate periods of time. Conversely, our mental attention increases when we can easily maintain fixation. Eye movements are the most basic visual ability (the eyes begin to move within the womb) and it is fair to assume that difficulty with eye movements generally precedes other visual problems. Interestingly, there is a growing body of evidence showing that decreased eye contact in the first two to six months of life may be the earliest sign of autism. Eye care practitioners who do not subscribe to the behavioral philosophy only evaluate eye movements briefly to determine if there is a damaged muscle. They are not concerned with the quality or sustainability of a person's eye movements.

Eye Teaming (binocularity) is important in order to have comfortable, efficient visual performance. We need our two eyes to point at the same thing at the same time. If the two eyes do not work together in a very precise and coordinated fashion, the result can be double vision. Double vision usually goes unreported by children even when they are asked directly if they ever see two of something they are looking at. There are several different types of eye teaming problems that can occur. In one common form, one eye may be turning in or out occasionally, frequently, or all of the time. Another common occurrence is for the image from one eye to be ignored by the brain because the images from the two eyes do not match well enough to combine into a single image. This may lead to what is known as a "lazy eye." Many of these eye teaming conditions are considered to be treatable surgically.

Most eye turns that disrupt efficient visual performance will go undetected without specialized testing because they are not cosmetically noticeable. Poor eye teaming can result in poor eye contact, frequent loss of place when reading, words appearing to move on the page, poor handwriting and/or other learning difficulties, headaches or eyestrain, etc. These complaints may appear in any combination. There will usually be an inability to stay at a visual task for any prolonged period of time, or at least an inability to sustain adequate performance for appropriate lengths of time. Poor eye teaming can also result in poor depth perception. This may contribute to poor general coordination, which can lead to dissatisfaction with or avoidance of activities such as riding a bicycle or playing sports. Some subtle eye teaming problems can actually cause more significant performance issues since the brain will continue the attempt to get both eyes working together. This can be especially true when the eye teaming deficiency is intermittent.

Focusing is another skill that is important for school, work, or sports performance. This skill allows rapid and accurate clarity as we look from one distance to another, such as looking from desk to chalkboard or hitting a tennis ball and then looking over at our opponent. It also permits clear focus at the various distances, especially the normal reading distance, for appropriate periods of time. Signs of a focusing problem may include blurred vision, fatigue or headaches while reading, and inability to see clearly (sometimes temporarily, sometimes permanently) at distance after reading. This may lead to a form of nearsightedness (an inability to see clearly in the distance without glasses or contact lenses) that is preventable if diagnosed properly and early. This type of nearsightedness is often reversible with proper and timely treatment.

Peripheral visual awareness is the foundation on which all visual skills and performance are built. It is the ability to be aware of, but not distracted by, the total available visual environment. This means that while attending to a specific object or task, we have the potential to keep a fairly large area (actually, a volume of space), and objects within that area, actively within our awareness without effort. Peripheral vision guides the eyes in locating precisely where they both should aim. This in turn allows the eyes to move smoothly together from one place to another, as well as giving information on where to focus so that the object will be clear. It provides considerable information about our surroundings and reduces the effort required to perform tasks and to move from one task to the next. Our peripheral vision lets us know about the size, shape, distance, and the speed and direction of movement of people and things around us. If all of this is not working smoothly and automatically, numerous problems are likely to result. Decreased peripheral awareness can lead to difficulty with reading, handwriting, and copying from the board, as well as reduced attention span, hyperactivity, fatigue, poor coordination, headaches, and some kinds of motion sickness. As you might expect, peripheral vision is critical for safe driving and successful participation in team sports.

Normal **visual acuity**, which we know as 20/20, is the ability to recognize a certain size letter at a certain distance. This is a measure of eyesight. While this is typically the main focus of most eye exams, in the overall scheme of visual performance it is not nearly as important as other aspects of visual function. Many people with 20/20 eyesight have significant visual development issues and/or inadequate visual skills that prevent high-level performance.

Visual development is important to acknowledge and to understand as well. All of the previous aspects of the visual process develop over time. In some cases, one or more aspects of visual development may be glossed over or poorly incorporated into overall performance. A person may function fairly well when there are such gaps in visual development, but they will use much more effort to perform visual tasks. Delayed or deficient visual development will likely result in a breakdown in visual performance and/or discomfort with normal and especially with more challenging visual demands.

In addition to the basic physical development of the human body within the womb, there is a functional side to the visual development story. It is known that there are eye movements within the womb. It is also known that peripheral vision is quite well developed at birth though we can only see details within arm's reach at birth and for some months after. Overall functional ability must continue to develop after we are born. This requires movement and a sufficiently stimulating visual environment. There are nerve cells in the brain that are only stimulated by light entering the right eye; there are other such cells that are only stimulated by light entering the left eye. More importantly, there are still other cells that are only stimulated when light is entering both eyes simultaneously. These cells are best stimulated when the two eyes are properly aligned. It was previously believed that all of these cells must be stimulated early in life if the brain is to have all the right "parts" or hardware with which to see and understand the visual environment. This belief has finally been debunked by the amazing story of a woman who came to be known as "Stereo Sue." She was given this name by renowned neurologist and author, Dr. Oliver Sacks.[1]

Stereo Sue is actually Susan Barry, PhD,[2] who developed stereo vision (the ability to see in 3-D) beginning in her late 40s. Dr. Barry is a professor of Biological Sciences and Neuroscience at Mount Holyoke College. In an attempt to align her crossed eyes, Dr. Barry had three eye muscle surgeries as a child on a total of five out of the 12 external eye muscles. Common medical wisdom continues even to this day, to misinterpret the Nobel Prize-winning research by David H. Hubel and Torsten Wiesel as saying that there is no ability for the brain to learn to use the two eyes in an integrated way if strabismus is present at an early age. Dr. Barry knew of the research and the beliefs held by surgeons when, in her late 40s she was told she could not possibly develop normal stereo vision, or depth perception, because of the early disruption to her visual system at or near birth. Dr. Barry was fortunate enough to find her way to Dr. Theresa Ruggiero who arranged an excellent vision therapy program. Dr. Barry's story is beautifully and expertly told in her book, *Fixing My Gaze: A Scientist's Journey into Seeing in Three Dimensions.*[6] The bottom line is that optometric vision therapy was able to accomplish what almost everyone in the medical community was certain could not be done. In fact, David Hubel confirmed Dr. Barry's achievement of high level stereo with vision therapy, encouraged her to publicize her story, and strongly endorsed her book. Dr. Barry's story has unfortunately not yet convinced most other eye care providers of what behavioral optometry has to offer. Dr. Barry continues to lecture to a variety of audiences, sharing her excitement about the changes she experienced in her visual process. You can even see her on You-Tube and TED Talks.

Scientists who study vision in order to know how we see understand that vision is a process of the brain, not just the eyes. In fact, the part of the eye that converts light into information and images is part of the brain. The eyes send direct signals to numerous parts of the brain and body. Many who study the brain focus their attention on one specific area of the brain devoted to seeing - the visual cortex. However, there are various pathways from the eyes to other parts of the brain involved in balance, stress responses, emotions, and other behavior. All of these areas are to some extent involved in the visual process, since information in many of these pathways travels in both directions. More connections are being discovered all the time.

The only concern of eye muscle surgeons is the cosmetic alignment of the eyes, not the overall function and development of the visual process.

Body posture is a critical factor in visual performance. When posture is other than optimal for a given task, there is a disturbance of visual performance. This disturbance can be temporary, or it may become permanent if these postural alterations persist. Studies have shown that the best way to improve or rehabilitate dysfunctional visual processing is to include movement of some or all of the body in the retraining process. These findings support the clinical experiences of countless behavioral optometrists over the years and the importance of the connections between posture, movement, and visual performance. This means that passive use of vision will not stimulate enhancement of overall function. Movement must be incorporated into the treatment process so that other nerve pathways are activated and stimulated simultaneously with the visual system in order to achieve the best results. This is due to the fact that the visual process is constantly integrating with other senses and other parts of the brain and body. Eye muscle surgery, to realign the eyes, simply ignores this research. These surgical procedures are simply used to cause the eyes to appear straight when viewed by others. There is absolutely no involvement of the person in this surgical process.

Most doctors who provide eye care either have no interest in the concepts described in this chapter or do not feel that they have any pertinence to the issue of vision as they see it. Again, it must be pointed out that the typical definition of vision is strictly a matter of eyesight, or visual acuity. Those who deal with vision as a more complex and dynamic process believe that ignoring these factors makes it difficult to achieve optimal visual performance. They feel that the highest level of care cannot be provided without addressing all the issues previously presented. This is one reason eye muscle surgery rarely provides any real improvement in overall visual function or development. The primary goal, in fact the only real goal, of eye muscle surgery is the cosmetic alignment of the eyes. It is not about the overall function and development of the visual process. Medical literature on the subject rarely even mentions high level binocularity and overall visual function as issues in regards to performing, and following up on, eye muscle surgery.

Chapter Two

WHY THINGS GO WRONG

There are various reasons for problems with visual function and a wide variety of visual conditions warranting specialized care. Here we will mostly be concerned with problems of eye teaming. Eye teaming problems can arise for many reasons. Most vision problems begin with visual development gaps or delays. There can also be problems related to improper use of the visual system and what we call visual stress. A.M. Skeffington, the original driving force behind behavioral optometry, starting in the 1930s, talked about the biologically unacceptable, socially compulsive near work that we all do every day from the time we enter school (if not sooner), often until we draw our final breath. What Skeffington meant was that our visual systems were not designed for the kind of close work we do so much of in modern culture - and it is getting to be more, not less so, with all the computers, iPhones, iPads, electronic readers, etc. 3-D movies are also causing vision related symptoms in a significant percentage of the population. Many people end up with complaints of eye fatigue, headaches, and even neck ache due to visual stress. These symptoms and the visual deficiencies causing them can be eliminated with proper lenses and vision therapy. Visual stress is not an issue with newborns and infants, but it is still an important aspect of visual function and dysfunction that warrants mentioning even for young children.

Clearly visual stress, as described above, is not causing eye teaming problems in the newborn and very young, but we want to make sure they have the best possible eye teaming skills before they attempt to read, write, and drive.

I have worked with many adults who can recall specific emotionally charged events in their lives that occurred just before their eye teaming problems were first noticed. One man in his 40s told me that he was hit in the head with a stick and suddenly developed intermittent double vision. This seemed plausible but not particularly likely based on his description of events. As we continued to work together over time, he started to remember things a little more clearly and eventually realized that this event occurred around the same time his parents separated, ultimately leading to their divorce. Other conditions which typically involve eye teaming problems include high fevers, seizures, cerebral palsy, Down Syndrome, autism, developmental delays, concussions and other traumatic brain injuries, strokes, etc. It is very rare, even in these situations for one or more of the eye muscles to be structurally unsound though there can be neurological damage, making treatment more challenging but still very worthwhile.

There are also cases where eye teaming problems appear at birth or in the first few months of life for reasons which remain unknown to this day. These are clearly not related to the kind of visual stress I just described. In any event, when things go wrong, adaptations must be made in order to function with some level of success and relative comfort. One possible adaptation is amblyopia (so-called lazy eye). This can happen if the brain decides its best bet is to try to ignore and stop using the eye that turns inappropriately. The eye turn might be intermittent at first, but if the problem persists and no better solution emerges, the brain might cause the eye to turn more often (and possibly farther) so that eventually the poor alignment becomes constant. The brain then stops depending on that eye for input and the eye stops receiving and transmitting reliable information. Of course this is really the brain's doing, but describing this becomes very cumbersome for our purposes.

There are those who feel that all visual conditions are genetically predetermined. However, there are numerous studies and countless clinical success stories that prove otherwise. Either way, there is tremendous potential for improvement in function given the opportunity and proper guidance. If heredity was such a clear indicator of visual conditions across generations, then identical twins would have identical conditions, and this is not necessarily the case. If eye problems were simply a matter of physical mechanisms, then there would not be people with multiple personality disorders whose visual (and other) conditions varied greatly when each of the various personalities surfaces. A damaged eye muscle will hinder the ability of the eye to move freely and properly in some or all directions. Even a faulty eye muscle, as seen in a condition called Brown's Syndrome, does not preclude a successful outcome - greater range of eye teaming - with vision therapy. All aspects of the visual process must be properly evaluated and addressed if a truly successful outcome is desired, even if there is a faulty eye muscle.

Some surgeons are now telling parents that there is nothing wrong with the child's eye muscle, but "that's how we fix it."

In all cases, eye muscle surgery results in a permanently damaged eye muscle. This includes muscles that were previously healthy. This is simply an unavoidable effect of surgery. I have had many parents come to me for a second opinion after their surgical consult, hoping to find a way to avoid surgery for their child. Some surgeons are now telling parents that "there is nothing wrong with the child's eye muscle, but that's how we fix it." Apparently some people find this scenario less than comforting and difficult to reconcile in their minds.

My dear colleague, mentor, and friend, Dr. Robert Kraskin, shared the following analogy with me. Think of the visual system as a plant. A healthy plant, growing unobstructed, will grow straight toward the light, maintaining a fairly straight, upright posture. If some obstruction is placed between the plant and the light, the plant will grow in some other direction, seeking out the light. It will attempt to find the most effective route to achieve its goal of unobstructed access to the light. However, once an obstruction is introduced and it starts bending and twisting toward the light, the plant is never quite the same. In more extreme cases, the structure of the plant may change so much that its very survival is jeopardized. Otherwise, it may survive, but may have a strange appearance and/or fragile structure. If the adaptive process of the obstructed plant seeking out the light is guided and properly supported, even its strange appearance can be handled in a way that will not interfere with its health and continued growth and development. The visual system experiences similar conditions, and our brains search for the easiest way to derive meaning and direct action.[4]

Here's a typical situation. A school aged child is seated in the classroom according to the first letter in his last name. The lighting and typical activity routine of the class cause the child to maintain an awkward posture to keep his eyes, mind, and body focused on what the teacher is doing. Remember, the visual system is intimately linked to the body and posture. It must adapt to less than optimal postural conditions in order to maintain an acceptable relationship between the visual system and the rest of the body, and perform effectively. The child returns to the same seat, day after day in most cases, which creates a habitual disturbance. The child in this new postural arrangement will find a way to stabilize and integrate everything in order to minimize the expenditure of energy. This occurs in different degrees for different people. In fact, some people have enough flexibility to maintain an acceptable level of performance without making any major or permanent adaptations.

These changes in visual behavior often become permanent because the person maintains their adaptations even though their situation has likely changed. This causes something like a structural change in the visual process to occur. Once this occurs, the visual system and the quality of visual performance are never quite the same. This is only one example of an obstruction of the visual system; there are many others. One quick note: I stated that the changes can become permanent. This may not be entirely accurate since these changes may simply become the foundation for future adaptation. They are also typically responsive to therapeutic lenses and vision therapy, both of which can help reverse negative adaptations and will be discussed in detail later.

Some eye teaming problems occur at or very shortly after birth.

In the past, it was commonly believed that some infants were born with crossed eyes. Some still hold to this concept, but most contend that in nearly all cases these conditions actually arise somewhat later, within the first few months of life. These infants have an obvious turning in of one or both eyes, and are quickly seen by an ophthalmologist in most cases. This is often important since some eye turns can be associated with serious, sometimes life-threatening

26

conditions. This type of situation is very rare, but it is surely better to rule this out and be on the safe side. It is also possible, although extremely rare, that one or more eye muscles may be damaged; this must also be determined. Eye muscle damage can occur during a forceps delivery. It is also possible that certain types of neurological damage can interfere with the function of an eye muscle. These types of problems are quite rare and are easily diagnosed. Once such problems have been ruled out, it can be safely assumed that the eye turn is strictly the result of a developmental/functional problem.

Most ophthalmologists will recommend a single strategy in all cases where a cosmetically noticeable eye turn is present. Ophthalmologists routinely prefer attempting to realign the eyes with eye muscle surgery, and that is likely the only option they will offer. Sometimes they will consider long-term patching or eye drop therapy before resorting to surgery. In addition, they will recommend eye muscle surgery without even a hint of need for any follow-up treatment, with the possible exception of another surgery. Again it should be said that ophthalmologists will easily recommend surgery even when they know full well that there is nothing wrong with any of the eye muscles. Most surgeons are convinced that there are no other options, so they are committed, in good conscience, to recommending surgery.

The cause of eye turns at such an early age remains uncertain. In fact, there are two opposing schools of thought that have been unable to reconcile their differences for over 100 years. One school holds that the muscles are at fault; this is not to say that there is muscle damage per se, but rather that the muscles are unable to coordinate their actions properly. I'm not sure how they think the eye muscles are supposed to coordinate their movements without instructions from the brain, but I will have to leave that discussion to the ophthalmologists.

Vision therapy helps an individual train the brain to use the eyes more efficiently.

The other school of thought contends that the brain is unable to coordinate the two eyes properly when there is an eye teaming problem in the absence of muscle damage. This would seem to be a critical factor in deciding whether or not surgery is the best option to pursue. Remember, it is very rare for there to be damaged eye muscles, even in newborns and infants with poor eye alignment. Most people with eye turns are able to move their eyes fully in all directions, which is the standard method of determining the presence or absence of a damaged muscle. Nonetheless, eye muscle surgery is done routinely in such cases. In most cases, surgery is performed in the absence of any other therapy. This makes it difficult for the brain to ever get the two eyes working comfortably and efficiently as a team. The eyes can only work well together when the brain has properly developed these skills. This is a problem of neurological development. Vision therapy can achieve this goal in most cases when the brain has not managed to do this on its own.

Think of what would happen if you injured any muscle in your body. You might need some sort of supportive device to assure that the muscle is stabilized and not subject to further injury while it heals. If the injury is bad enough, you might need an operation to repair the damage. In either case you would expect to need some rehabilitative program to return the muscle to its pre-injury state of health, since it was out of use for some period of time. Whenever a muscle is damaged, it has a negative effect on other muscles that depend on it to function normally. Various other muscles will be out of operation during the time the damaged muscle must heal. All the involved muscles will then need therapy, once the time is right, to return things to as normal a state as possible.

An eye muscle that is surgically altered will sustain a significant decrease in its range and flexibility of movement.

Those who perform eye muscle surgeries typically do not see the need for any therapy to assure that the eye muscles will be returned to their best possible state after an operation. This would seem to be further evidence that there was never actually anything wrong with the muscles to begin with, at least not before the surgery. Surgery, by its very nature, must do some damage to the muscle that had the surgery while attempting the desired outcome. There is a significant decrease in the normal flexibility and range of movement of an eye muscle once it has been surgically altered. Each surgery further diminishes the effectiveness of the muscle. I examined one woman who had undergone 10 eye muscle surgeries - I'm not sure how many surgeries were done on any individual muscle. Colleagues have reported seeing people who had even more eye muscle surgeries than that.

We now know that there are very special muscle fibers that communicate vital information from the eye muscle to the brain. These specialized fibers happen to reside in the exact area where the eye muscle is severed during eye muscle surgery. These very special and critical fibers, known as Felderstruktur fibers, are certainly damaged during the eye muscle surgery. These fibers cannot repair themselves, and new ones cannot be created.[6] This is even more reason to follow all eye muscle surgery with vision therapy, to help the brain figure out how to use the now-modified equipment.

Most eye teaming problems result from less than optimal visual development and/or improper use of the visual system. Cosmetically realigning an eye surgically does nothing to address the fundamental issues involved, which is a major reason re-operation is so common.

Eye teaming problems mostly result from a person's need to modify visual behavior in response to visual demands. Visual stress results when a person's natural response to daily visual demands is less than optimal. Visual stress is essentially any situation where the individual's ability to apply their visual process comfortably and effectively is overpowered by the demands of the task. This could be a fleeting, rarely occurring problem or one that is chronic. The response is likely to be chronic if the difficulty is also chronic. Chronic stress will cause an adaptation that becomes "structured in." That means it is likely to become a permanent part of all visual performance. This often happens even though the adaptation is only useful for a specific task and it may actually interfere with optimal performance of many other tasks.

Add in the very likely postural aspect and you have a systemic alteration of structure and function. When postural adaptations cause the body to be improperly aligned, the brain senses this imbalance and takes measures to reconcile the visual system with the rest of the body.

It may be too late for the adaptation to change easily once the setting created in response to stress or ineffective performance is maintained. That is, unless there is intervention with therapeutic lenses and/or vision therapy.

Since these problems typically persists for a considerable period of time, the adaptation will persist until there is some consistency throughout the visual system and the body. These adaptations assure that the eyes are coordinating with the rest of the body. The only problem is that this new arrangement is one of necessity, not efficiency. It may provide better performance of certain specific tasks, but it can often lead to decreased general performance over time. At best, such adaptations can be useful for certain circumstances, but rarely as an overall way of meeting the wide variety of visual demands we all face. The adaptations tend to become habitual patterns that permeate all of our activities and therefore are likely to become a kind of new default setting. That is, unless there is intervention with therapeutic lenses and/or vision therapy. If these adaptations become habitual they can lead to undesirable permanent changes in visual performance. This can lead to nearsightedness, astigmatism, and/or more difficult visual problems such as lazy eye (amblyopia) or various types of eye teaming problems including strabismus.

We can be fairly sure that a person with undesirable visual findings has undergone some type of visual stress and has adapted in order to continue functioning at some acceptable level.

One difficulty in the treatment of most functional visual problems is that the treatment is usually focused on the signs and symptoms, not the cause. Generally, visual conditions and symptoms that are evidenced during an evaluation are seen as the thing to be treated or eliminated. This philosophy is lacking on several levels. Actually, the condition that becomes obvious enough to propel us to the doctor due to symptoms and complaints is not the true problem. Any such complaints, symptoms, or conditions are actually indications of the person's response to the original problem, which is related to the difficulty maintaining adequate performance in the face of normal, everyday visual demands.

Think of the twists and turns in the shape of the plant discussed earlier; we do not always see the factors that caused the plant to grow in a way that is other than straight and strong. However, with experience we can be fairly sure that a plant with an unusual growth pattern relative to other members of its species has undergone some type of stress and has adapted in order to survive. We can be fairly sure that a person with undesirable visual findings has undergone some type of visual stress and adapted in order to continue functioning at some acceptable level. With a plant, we can determine if the soil is poor, if there is obstructed lighting, or if there is some other problem; then we can correct the problem. With a person, we can thoroughly evaluate their visual status once to have a reasonable idea as to where the problem started and how to improve performance and set future development of the visual process on a better course.

Chapter Three

WHERE DO I TURN FOR HELP?

It is always heartbreaking to realize that your child has a health issue requiring treatment. The mere presence of such a condition is difficult enough. Next comes the decision regarding what to do about it. Can we just leave it alone? Will she outgrow it? Is there any way to fix it? Can we somehow deal with this on our own, or do we need to seek professional help? Who is the best person to consult once the decision to do something is made.

Strabismus could seem to be merely a cosmetic problem, or there could be noticeable difficulty associated with the eye teaming issues. There could be global developmental delays and/or learning related difficulties related to poor visual development. Many people with strabismus experience double vision, clumsiness, poor coordination, fatigue related to visually demanding work such as reading or computer related activities, headaches, or vague discomfort seemingly unrelated to the visual process.

Visual development and overall development are intimately linked.

An infant or very young child may show signs of overall developmental delays. This is quite common with children whose eyes are noticeably misaligned. In fact, most children diagnosed with developmental problems have eye teaming and tracking problems and/or other visual development issues. These visual problems can be severe or more subtle, but they are likely to interfere with general development due to the tremendous importance of the visual process in our lives. Proper diagnosis and treatment of these visual problems almost always result in significant improvement in overall development.

Dozens of studies (outside the field of optometry) over the past few years have shown a strong relationship between eye movements/eye contact and the presence of autism spectrum disorders (ASDs). One study showed that infants later diagnosed with ASDs exhibited declines in eye fixation from 2 to 6 months of age. This pattern is not observed in infants who do not develop ASD. Every child exhibiting autism spectrum behaviors should be evaluated by a behavioral optometrist. Many of these children have visual development delays that respond well to vision therapy and therapeutic lenses.

The age of the person when the problem is first noticed might have bearing on the outcome as well as the possible interventions. It tends to be easier to treat a problem that is picked up early. While it can often be challenging to work with very young children, the rewards are too great simply to give up or to delay treatment because it may be difficult. If you end up in the office of a doctor who says your child is too young to benefit from vision therapy, keep looking. Most behavioral optometrists have experience with infants and very young children and are willing to do the difficult work necessary to evaluate and treat developmental visual conditions. It took a number of years in practice before I began working with very young children and infants, but once I started, I found it very rewarding and consistently successful.

It is important, in most cases, to begin therapy as early as possible if only to prevent adaptations from becoming more permanently influential in the child's development and behavior. One of the benefits of vision therapy and developmental lenses is the disruption of patterns within the visual process, which when left unchanged, tend to become structured-in. Such structured-in behavior patterns become the norm unless and until an outside influence is brought to bear. The short-term goal for the youngest patients is sometimes nothing more than making sure the less-than-desirable adaptations cannot get a foot-hold. The hope is always to do more than this, but if that is all that's available at the time, it is still worthwhile. This will at least set the stage for later on, when the child is capable of benefitting from more thorough vision therapy.

Behavioral optometrists have had many decades of success helping children to keep these less than optimal adaptations from becoming permanent. This is important when looking at the big picture. Success is more likely if the visual system is kept flexible by introducing vision therapy and therapeutic lenses as early as possible even if the bulk of the therapy must wait until the child is older and easier to work with. Vision therapy has a long history of helping people of all ages with many types of visual development issues.

In some ways it is more difficult for adults to make changes in behaviors to which they have grown accustomed and structured-in to everything they do over the years. However, adults have the advantage of knowing what they want and need. Adults tend to be more motivated because they can intellectually understand their deficits and how these deficits are impacting their lives, in ways that are typically unavailable to young children. The interaction of all the factors must be considered, but just as it is never too early to start, it is never too late to try. The current age range of my patients is 2 to 86.

The cosmetic appearance of a child with an eye turn is certainly something every parent wants to eliminate. Even though this is the most obvious aspect of the condition, it is not the most significant issue.

It is obviously stressful when a parent discovers that their newborn, young infant or child appears to have an eye turn. This misalignment may appear to happen occasionally, frequently, or constantly. Few things are more emotionally charged than discovering a problem with an infant. An understandably concerned parent will quickly seek an expert who can explain the problem and advise treatment. The unusual cosmetic appearance is certainly something every parent wants to eliminate. It is important to realize that even though this is the most obvious aspect of the condition, it is not the most significant issue. The focus of professionals should be on the overall function and development of the visual process whenever there is such an obvious eye-teaming problem. Consistent integration between the two eyes, which is only possible when the brain is operating both inputs (eyes) effectively, is the best and safest way to get and keep the eyes straight. The importance of a smoothly operating visual system cannot be overemphasized.

Ophthalmologists

As mentioned previously, there are two main approaches to dealing with eye teaming problems. One group of experts that assesses and treats such problems is ophthalmologists, medical doctors specializing in eye diseases and medical treatments. These treatments typically involve drugs and/or surgery. Ophthalmologists usually decide to operate in order to make the eyes look straight when the eye turn is cosmetically noticeable. They typically believe that eye muscle surgery is the only solution.

Unfortunately, making the eyes appear straight does not always assure that they will function the way they are supposed to. In fact, making the eyes look straight is not even a guarantee that they will remain straight. A significant percentage of eye muscle surgeries last less than five years. The eyes will lose the surgical alignment over time, which often leads to further surgery to realign them.[8-11] Some experts feel that such a surgery has been successful if the eyes appear straight at any time after the operation.[1] This means that if the eyes appear straight even for a very brief time, that is good enough for the surgeon. This is probably not good enough for the anxious parent and is certainly not good enough for the developing infant or child.

Compensating lenses rarely have positive long-term effects on the visual process. It is necessary to change visual habits and behaviors with vision therapy to achieve optimal, lasting improvement.

Lenses will sometimes be prescribed to attempt to straighten crossed eyes. In these cases, there is believed to be a focusing problem that contributes to the eyes being crossed. Lenses may help the eyes appear to straighten, and the eyes may look straight when the lenses are being worn under these conditions. However, when the lenses are removed, the eyes will immediately cross again. One reason for this is the fact that such lenses are designed to compensate for a focusing problem believed to be a cause or the cause of the eye turn. Compensating lenses such as these rarely have any significant positive long-term effects on the visual process, especially when used without vision therapy. Compensating lenses rarely affect the kinds of internal changes that result from vision therapy. These lenses essentially do the work that the brain needs to learn to do for itself in a more effective way than what it has been doing up to that time. Because of this, the long-term effects of compensating lenses are more likely to weaken the visual system than strengthen it. There is greater likelihood of long-term improvement with therapeutic/developmental lenses (as discussed in Chapter five) and vision therapy designed to help the person modify their visual patterns.

Prisms may also be used as compensating lenses. The purpose of compensating prism is essentially to trick the brain into thinking both eyes are pointing at the same place at the same time. This typically has the same effect as lenses that deal with the focusing aspect. They may work while they are being worn, but take them off and the eyes jump back to where they were. Again, this approach has the prisms doing the work the brain is not yet managing to do. Compensating prisms also have the added risk of the brain adapting to them, which often results in the need for stronger and stronger prisms over time because the eye turn keeps worsening. Vision therapy is likely to lead to more permanent improvement and the need for weaker prisms or preferably no prisms at all.

Another frequently used approach is to patch (sometimes using an adhesive patch, especially in the youngest patients) the "good" eye for long periods, forcing the "bad" eye to work more. This approach has been scientifically proven to be mediocre at best. Patching can be helpful if done properly, but passively wearing a patch for days, weeks, or months at a time is cruel and does not work. There sometimes is improvement in eyesight if the patch is worn in this way, but that improvement is usually short lived. Some doctors (including some behavioral optometrists) are now, instead of a patch, using drugs (eye drops) that paralyze the focusing of the "good" eye, making that eye unusable during normal activities for as long as the drops are in effect. Either way, this can be quite debilitating for the child and is not something I would ever include in my therapy program. Most children will do anything to remove the patch; in response some doctors splint the young child's arms so they cannot pull the patch off with their hands. Some children have learned to defeat even this seemingly foolproof attempt to control them by rubbing their faces against some object in order to scrape off the patch. Obviously, there is no way for a child to get around the eye drop method other than waiting for the drug's effects to wear off.

Besides all of this, there is one fundamental flaw to both compensating lenses/prisms and this type of patching or drug intervention (all known as penalization therapy); their goal is to provide an external device that will "correct" the problem of the eye turning. The flaw lies in the fact that, as brought out earlier, the turning eye is not the actual problem. The inappropriately turning eye is usually just the outward appearance of the less obvious underlying problem.

The real problem is a mismatch in visual information processing. This means that there is a miscommunication within the brain. The brain is not accurately interpreting the visual information coming in from the environment and is unable properly to integrate the way the two eyes coordinate. Therefore the brain cannot send accurate instructions to the eyes about where and how to aim as a team. Briefly, the brain is not accurately assessing the distance, direction, and spatial properties of external objects and the overall environment. This concept of mismatching is part of the root cause of most functional visual problems. The eyes work according to the directions they receive from the brain.

The application of external devices, or crutches, will not serve to change the way the brain processes information, and therefore will not change visual behavior in a way that will achieve the optimal benefit, which is continued development sufficient to meet the changing needs that confront us as we move through life. Such lenses and patching techniques should not, however, be confused with the quite strategic use of lenses, and possibly a more strategic approach to patching, with a developmental/ behavioral optometric approach. It is not the devices themselves that are appropriate or inappropriate, it is the way in which they are used that can be a blessing or a problem. Most optometrists do not practice with a developmental/behavioral approach and subscribe to the same philosophy as ophthalmologists when assessing and treating eye teaming conditions. Behavioral optometrists use lenses and patches very differently from other doctors, and the results are very different.

The eyes act according to instructions they receive from the brain. Lenses will only help in changing the way the brain processes information, and therefore changing visual behavior in a way that will achieve the optimal benefit, when they are derived and utilized based on a developmentally oriented philosophy.

Behavioral Optometrists

The other main group of experts is *behavioral* or *developmental* optometrists who are doctors of optometry most of whom have pursued post-doctoral education in treating developmental and functional vision conditions such as eye teaming problems. The primary focus of ophthalmologists and most optometrists is clear eyesight. They are likely to miss a subtle eye turn problem. They are mainly interested in straightening the eye as a strictly mechanical process when there is a cosmetically noticeable eye turn.

On the other hand, a behavioral optometrist evaluates a person's visual status in order to understand how that person has been using the tremendous potential of the visual process to direct action while engaged in normal everyday activities. How is that person using the visual process to meet their current needs, and how can the efficiency of the visual process be enhanced going forward, to meet the changing, usually increasing demands to come? This is achieved by doing an evaluation that is designed to identify and understand the adaptations that person is using to compensate for the less than adequate use of the visual process. It is also important to determine how lenses might help stimulate visual development to move in a better direction.

Behavioral optometrists rarely use drugs and never use surgery to bring about changes in eye teaming performance. Their understanding of the processes of visual development and performance is the foundation for very different philosophies and approaches to vision care. Behavioral optometrists are experienced in using vision therapy and developmental lenses, which are noninvasive approaches for enhancing visual performance.

As stated above, behavioral optometrists will typically use lenses, prisms, and selective eye patching within the context of a dynamic, interactive vision therapy program. The difference is that behavioral optometrists are more likely to use lenses to achieve more dramatic, more comprehensive, longer lasting (usually permanent) results. It is also important to note that these lenses are not intended to compensate. They are designed to stimulate the brain in particular ways so that desirable changes in visual habits and behaviors are more likely to occur. The changes resulting from therapeutic lenses and vision therapy emerge from the inside out, rather than being a passive response to a device that does the work itself, treating the brain as more innocent bystander than active participant.

Patching should only be used under specific, controlled conditions to maximize the beneficial effects while greatly reducing the adverse effects. Full time patching is still considered (by some) to be a treatment of choice for many eye teaming problems. Research by Crewther, SG & Crewther, Mitchell, DE[12] beginning in the 1970s has shown that this approach is neither dynamic enough nor successful enough to warrant continued support. It is also known that full time patching can actually *cause* problems with the normal development of the visual process. This is especially important to consider with infants and children up to the age of 7 or so, since there is danger of interfering with proper development of brain cells related to the patched eye as well as the development of cells that need both eyes to be stimulated simultaneously for proper development. This, of course, is the very population that tends to be treated with either the adhesive eye patch or the blurring drops - the two things that are most likely to cause problems in this way.

In addition, there are social/emotional issues with wearing a patch in public. Children are not always sophisticated in their ability to deal with someone who looks or acts differently. Children wearing eye patches are often subjected to teasing by their peers and may feel alienated. I have never found it necessary to have a child wear a patch in public. There are occasions when I assign some home activities during which a patch is worn, but I've never had a child wear a patch outside the home, except in my office where everyone is likely to wear a patch at one time or another.

The concepts and practices of behavioral optometry are not so well known to the public. One problem that arises when a parent seeks advice from a variety of experts is that they get a variety of recommendations which are, in some cases, utterly different from one another though all seem to make sense when they are presented. This causes great confusion, and can, all too often, lead to a poor decision. I have seen many parents who felt they failed their child by opting for surgery. I never blame a parent for making such a decision; I blame the doctor who failed to properly inform the parent of all the available options. Behavioral optometric concepts are similarly unfamiliar to and poorly understood by many other professionals as well. This means that the average person seeking advice will very likely not be informed about all the available alternatives.

Another problem is that many of these experts have severe biases and prejudices against the behavioral optometric approach. This exists for a variety of reasons. One reason is that these professionals are not taught, nor are they interested in, behavioral/developmental approaches, so they dismiss them out of hand. They will claim that there is no scientific proof that these "eye exercises" (as they call them) can have any effect on how the eyes work. This claim is nothing more than an opinion and cannot be supported by any actual evidence, scientific or otherwise.

In fact, more and more science supports the theories and practices of behavioral optometry. Unfortunately, the contrary position continues to be held very firmly by many who are looked to as experts, and they tend to put forth their opinions as though they were facts. It is hard not to heed these recommendations, especially when they are put forth with such certainty. It is best to go into any important treatment program with healthy skepticism. This is especially true for one that may be new to you. One important fact remains: surgery is irreversible. Vision therapy and lens therapy are totally noninvasive with no known negative side effects. The only likely effects of vision therapy are improvement in visual development, performance, and comfort.

One important thing to remember is that you have the final word in your decision making process. It is much more difficult to make the best decision if you have incomplete information about the available options. You can only decide based on what is available to you at the time. The main purpose of this book is to provide more information to help you make the best decision possible based on all known factors causing these problems to arise, as well as all the available approaches to solving the problems.

There are thousands of behavioral optometrists throughout the United States and across the world. As with all health care providers, there are various approaches taken by different practitioners. The core concepts throughout the behavioral optometric community are pretty much the same, but each practitioner has his or her own unique style. This is as it should be since we are dealing with human beings on both sides of the process. A one-size-fits-all approach will not be effective in a dynamic and human process like vision therapy. Behavioral optometry requires that the practitioner be flexible and innovative in order to deal with whatever twists and turns present themselves in the course of dealing with any individual that requests our participation in their healing process.

It is important, when choosing a doctor to diagnose and/or treat a problem with eye alignment, to ask the right questions. Most people are anxious in the doctor's office and often forget to ask all the questions they came in with. Doctors can sometimes have difficulty communicating all possible options regarding a particular case when face-to-face with their patient. This is not necessarily a character flaw. Specialists see conditions which are unusual or frightening to the average person on a routine basis. These conditions are commonplace to them so they may lose sight of just how taken aback the patient or parent might feel or what level of understanding there may be. In some cases, doctors do not feel it is important for a patient to know all the issues. The thinking is that the doctor will take care of everything, and the patient must trust, sit back, and let the doctor do whatever needs to be done. Therefore, it is absolutely necessary for the average individual to be as informed as possible before walking into such a situation. Even doctors can make these mistakes when waking into another doctor's office as a patient.

There are several important questions to have ready when trying to select a doctor to help with visual problems. You will want to have these questions answered before deciding whether or not to proceed with strabismus surgery, and in order to know that you are working with the right doctor:

- **Is there an alternative to surgery in any case of an eye that turns inappropriately?**

- **If surgery is indicated, how likely is it that one operation will be all that is needed?**

- **Will the eyes remain totally straight after surgery, and for how long?**

- **How will surgery affect the way the eyes work as a team?**

- **Should there be some type of therapy after the surgery?**

- **Will surgery improve visual function and eliminate all visual complaints?**

- **Is there actually damage to one or more eye muscles?**

- **What level of depth perception is present at this time?**

- **What level of depth perception should be expected after the surgery?**

- **What are the criteria for a successful surgery?**

- **How often will there be reevaluations, and over what length of time?**

- **Is surgery appropriate even though my child's eye only loses alignment some of the time?**

- **Is surgery appropriate even though it is not always the same eye that turns?**

There are also various issues that should be addressed during the evaluation. It should raise suspicion that the style of care being offered may not be what you are looking for if these issues are not addressed. With eye teaming problems, it would be very unusual if there were no other issues besides cosmetic appearance that are of concern. Responses to the following questions should come out at some point during the first visit:

Have you ever experienced any of the following?

- Eyes tire easily or hurt
- Frequent headaches
- Eyes frequently red
- Double vision
- Closing or covering one eye
- Holding reading close
- Tilting head while reading
- Losing place while reading
- Pointing to keep place on page
- Words moving on page
- Poor reading comprehension
- Focus changes while reading
- Getting drowsy while reading
- Purposely avoiding reading
- Difficulty completing work on time
- Reversing letters/numbers
- Difficulty with spelling
- Poor handwriting skills

- Short attention span

- Blurry vision far away or close up

- Slow focusing from near to far or far to near

- Discomfort during or after computer work

- General developmental delays with talking, walking, social interaction, etc.

- Poor general coordination

- Motion sickness

- Sensitivity to light

Obviously, some of these issues deal with older children or adults as opposed to infants or very young children. All of these problems are possible for someone with an eye teaming problem. It is not likely that anyone would have all of these problems, but it would be quite unusual for such a person not to have experienced at least one or more of these at some point. If this is the case, elimination of these issues must be considered as a primary goal of any intervention, whether or not it includes surgery. Optimal visual function is of the utmost importance to a person's ability to achieve in our culture. There is no question that a person's appearance is an important issue. When someone does not look normal, it can be a significant obstacle in our culture as well. However, the inability to gather visual information effectively and comfortably is a tremendous handicap to making the most out of our learning, earning, and recreational opportunities. It is also important to understand that the brain's ability to operate the visual process efficiently is necessary for the eyes to appear straight and to stay that way.

Chapter Four

VISION THERAPY

Optometric vision therapy has been practiced since the 1930s across the United States. It is now widely practiced and sought after throughout Europe, Australia, and other parts of the world. Vision therapy is a program of activities designed to provide the appropriate conditions under which people can begin to understand how their visual process works, and how it can work better. By working better I mean that things we do every day will be done with less effort, greater efficiency, and with greater comfort and endurance. We are typically unaware of many of the subtleties of how our visual system is functioning as we go through our daily activities unless there are disruptions so obvious that we cannot avoid thinking about them. Strabismus is of course one of these disruptions for many people with the condition.

Most people don't associate their complaints with the visual process. Many people who suffer from headaches, fatigue, dry eyes, reading difficulties, poor coordination, and motion sickness have been helped with lenses and vision therapy. Many of these people were unaware that these issues were rooted in a poorly developed and poorly functioning visual system and sought help for other reasons. They were able to put all the pieces of the puzzle together and begin to plot a new path forward after their symptoms and complaints were discussed in the proper context as part of a thorough visual evaluation. Vision therapy is very likely needed when these kinds of complaints and symptoms have been allowed to continue for some period of time. Vision therapy has a very high success rate when deficits in the visual process are at the root of the problems.

Vision therapy is an interactive process designed to train the brain to use the eyes more efficiently. Remember, it is extremely rare for an eye muscle to be damaged. This is even true of an eye that appears crossed or turned out most or all of the time. Many parents who seek me out after getting a surgical consult, say that the surgeon told them there was nothing wrong with the child's eye muscles, but the way it is fixed is with eye muscle surgery. The surgeons are correct that in most cases there is nothing wrong with the eye muscles, but most of them ignore the fact that the visual process develops over the course of a lifetime and can be enhanced through vision therapy. Strabismus can be eliminated with vision therapy for a significant number of people, regardless of age.

The visual process involves many parts of the brain in an intricate web of nerve pathways going from the optic nerve at the back of the eye to over a dozen locations in many parts of the brain that we would not typically associate with vision. This includes areas of the brain involved with balance, movement, emotions, social interactions and language. There is integration between various functional components of brain activity and messages traveling to and from almost every part of the body. The eye muscles themselves are uniquely structured and very strong, yet very delicate.

At times during the vision therapy process, it can be useful to have a person try to be aware of feeling the movement of their eyes while doing certain activities. Many people find this very difficult at first because the eye muscles are such small muscles and because we are not typically attuned to feeling specific parts of our bodies, large or small, in action except when there is something wrong. Sometimes the ability to consciously tune into the movement of the eye muscles helps a person begin to change a habitual pattern that is holding them back. Eye movement training is a critical part of any vision therapy program whether or not the person can manage some level of conscious awareness of how the eyes are moving. The goal is for eye movements to be accurate, effortless, and unnoticed during normal daily activities.

Vision therapy is at its best when it involves using the visual process in a way that involves as much of the brain and body as possible. There exists a critical two-way relationship between movement and the visual process. Movement is essential for visual development and development in general and the primary purpose of the visual process is directing our movements, whether it be guiding our eyes across a page, guiding our hand as we write, clicking our mouse on a particular item on a computer screen, tapping out a text message or playing any kind of sport.

Vision therapy is an intricate process designed to involve an individual in his or her own healing process. A good vision therapy program will very likely include special lenses to stimulate brain development. Lenses often play a crucial role in vision improvement and can also be used to prevent visual difficulties from arising.

Eye muscle surgery places a person in a passive position - few things make us more passive than general anesthesia - while someone else performs a procedure which, it is claimed, will fix the problem. It seems clear that those who adhere to the mechanical/surgical philosophy are quite unfamiliar with, if not disinterested in, the issues and conditions that lie at the root of most eye teaming (and other) developmental/functional visual problems. The cavalier willingness to operate on eye muscles that are admittedly not damaged in any way would seem to prove this point. All this implies that most surgeons tend to be unfamiliar with exactly what the problem is, other than a cosmetic one. Those who subscribe to the developmental/behavioral philosophy of the visual process understand that the so-called "problem" is not the actual problem at all. Most symptoms, including strabismus, are signs of the person's attempts to function more easily.

This strange sounding idea might need some explanation. This was mentioned earlier, but bears repeating. Most visual problems result from a difficulty in dealing with processing visual information from the environment. In most cases, this is the result of gaps or delays in visual development. The brain must and will attempt to find a more effective way of dealing with its difficulty in managing the visual demands of normal daily life. Since most of us are unaware of the intricacies of the visual process, we make those attempts to function more effectively with little or no knowledge of what the best way to proceed might be. This is a normal part of the process of visual development, but sometimes we need to change a particular area of behavior to compensate for a weakness. This adaptation is likely to cause unintended repercussions in various aspects of performance.

The crossed eye is not the real problem. The real problem is the brain's inability to integrate and coordinate the two eyes. Realigning an eye only addresses the symptom - a cosmetic abnormality. Vision therapy is the best way to keep the eyes straight and working together.

The findings that emerge from any evaluation of the visual process paint a picture of the individual's attempts to come to terms with visual demands in everyday life. This basically provides an understanding of what has already happened up to that point in time. The simplest example of this is nearsightedness. A person diagnosed with nearsightedness is typically told that the problem is that they are nearsighted. This is like telling someone diagnosed with heart problems secondary to poor diet and lack of exercise that they have a faulty heart. They probably weren't born with a faulty heart, but the heart was damaged as a result of lifestyle. The lifestyle leading to the heart problem is the root cause of the outward issue. Post-surgical counseling for a change in lifestyle would be much more helpful to the individual than simply trying to repair the heart, and in fact modern medicine now recognizes the importance of diet and lifestyle regarding healthy heart function.

Most cases of nearsightedness are, at least in part, the result of lifestyle issues. Repeated ineffective attempts to manage the strain on the visual system inherent in close work frequently contribute to the emergence and/or worsening of nearsightedness. This means that the nearsightedness is not the root problem, but the result of adaptations and compensations in response to visual stress, and therefore a secondary issue. The trigger is the lack of an effective strategy for managing visually challenging tasks. Effective visual abilities are expected to develop through the normal course of events in our early years, but this does not always happen. In addition, close work in our modern culture is visually challenging because it is biologically unnatural, essentially unavoidable, and usually done for hours on end, day after day. This leads to any number of adaptive strategies, the most common of which is nearsightedness. Many eye teaming problems, tracking deficiencies, and focusing difficulties result from similar delays in visual development.

A common scenario: Johnny is born into a normal family and spends his early years in a normal home and school environment. Unbeknownst to everyone, Johnny has visual developmental delays that create difficulty with sustaining near work like reading, writing, and working at the computer. Johnny may notice that there is some sort of difficulty, but usually he will not, other than realizing that seeing far away is blurry or possibly knowing that he does not like to read. At some point Johnny becomes symptomatic and ends up at the eye doctor. If that doctor is a behavioral optometrist, there will be a thorough evaluation. The evaluation will likely generate some understanding of how things went wrong and how to move in a more positive direction from that point forward. If the doctor is not a behavioral optometrist, the symptoms will be treated, but the cause/response dynamic will not change. Johnny will continue to use his visual system the way he always has, and the symptoms are likely to return—if they ever went away. This is an all too common scenario for nearsighted children and the compensating glasses that enable clear distance sight almost always compound the deeper problem.

There are, unfortunately, cases where an infant is born with a turned (usually crossed) eye or develops an eye turn within the first few years of life. This is known as congenital (appearing at birth) or infantile (appearing within the first year of life) strabismus. These forms of strabismus are clearly not the result of excessive close work. They can still be successfully treated with lenses and/or vision therapy in a majority of cases. I have worked with numerous children between the ages of 2 and 4 with crossed eyes. Most of these children ended up with straight eyes that worked together properly, but more importantly, eyes that the brain was able make use of in an integrated way. Also, there was no need for risky surgeries.

One of the most important factors favoring vision therapy over surgery is the fact that in vision therapy, the individual is actively engaged in their own healing process, instead of being a passive subject. The doctor or therapist acts as a guide through the vision therapy process. All of the actual work is done by the person who stands to benefit from the process. Many people are searching for alternatives to standard medical practice for healing many types of ailments or injuries. Vision therapy stands as a complementary approach to standard medically oriented approaches since it requires a true partnership between practitioner and patient.

It is still possible to achieve positive results in children who are, shall we say, not overly enthusiastic about their vision therapy program. These children must actively participate in the therapy activities, even if they are not putting all their effort into it. The more engaged and interested a person is in their process of change, the better (or at least faster) the results are likely to be, but even the most disinterested will improve if they are at least minimally engaged in the vision therapy activities asked of them.

Vision therapy addresses the causes of visual difficulty, not merely the symptoms. Vision therapy is an interactive process that involves conscious attention and provides immediate feedback thereby stimulating new behavior patterns in the brain.

Vision therapy is an individualized program of activities that provides conditions for observation, practice, learning, and understanding of how we use the visual process. Each activity arranges the conditions that make it possible to utilize the various aspects of the visual process and visual performance in an appropriate and controlled environment. It is important to have a knowledgeable observer and guide during this process in order to monitor the many aspects of each activity and the progress over time. This will maximize the benefits from the vision therapy process and help assure the best final outcome. Some of the things that should be monitored are: breathing, posture, accuracy of performance, effects of lenses, and any changes in awareness of these things, etc.

There are now a number of computer programs that can be useful in improving visual performance. It is my opinion that a computer program pales in comparison to an in-office vision therapy program that involves movement, therapeutic lenses, and a behavioral optometrist (or possibly an experienced vision therapist) personally involved in all aspects of the therapy program. A truly good therapist (I have chosen to be doctor and therapist in my office) will be able to provide and help each person experience feedback during each vision therapy activity. A good therapist knows how to make the most out of "mistakes" that occur. I tell my patients that my job is to create a safe environment where they are free to make mistakes; their job is to make as many mistakes as necessary to complete the task as best they can. A computer cannot take advantage of a teachable moment, when something happens that helps bring about a breakthrough. There are no teachable moments possible with surgery.

Movement, as mentioned earlier, is a critical aspect of a good vision therapy program. Movement is necessary for normal human development. Movement is also necessary for normal visual development. Don't forget, the primary purpose of the visual process is to direct action. Movement and the visual process are inseparable. It stands to reason, then, that a vision therapy program designed to improve visual performance and visual development should involve movement. By movement I do not mean moving a mouse or a joystick. I mean moving the body and doing real physical activities that have direct and immediate consequences in the real world. Examples include walking on a specially designed walking rail with special glasses, hitting a ball suspended from the ceiling, doing fine motor activities with different lenses, and coordinating various body movements such as hopping, skipping, or tumbling. All of these are of course visually guided actions requiring awareness of self and spatial awareness of one's surroundings.

Acuvision 1000

I have a wall-mounted electronic touch-screen that displays one one-inch diameter lighted target at a time (Figure 1). The goal is to hit each target as quickly as possible, which causes the next target to appear. The targets can be programmed to appear in sequence or randomly located. A variety of speed settings are available so that the length of time each target is displayed can be changed as

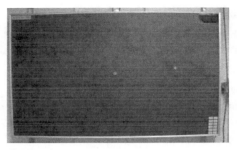

Figure 1.

desired. This unit is no longer being produced but there are other similar devices available.

This is an activity that has something for everyone. First, it is typically done in a standing position and requires direct eye/hand integration. I like this procedure because it involves standing, movement, eye/hand coordination, peripheral awareness and reaction time. Smaller children will have more of a tendency to look at each target rather than relying on peripheral vision, but this still provides some quality interaction. The procedure can also be done using red/green filters so that only one eye can see the target while both eyes are able to see everything else. This has been especially helpful in strabismus cases since it is common for people with strabismus to use one eye more than the other. This procedure is very good for helping the brain better connect the lesser-used eye with the rest of the body.

Pegboard Rotator

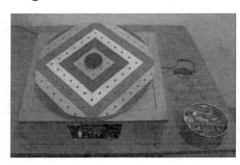

Figure 2.

The pegboard rotator (Figure 2) is a commonly used piece of equipment in vision therapy. I typically have people do this using one eye at a time. I also have them wear two different pairs of lenses - first, lenses that require an increase in near focusing, and then lenses that relax the focusing system. These lenses (all lenses in fact, other than contact lenses) change not only the focusing demand, but also where things appear to be in space, that is, how far away they appear.

Here are the instructions: "Take one peg and hold it near your chin. Pick a hole to aim for and look right into that hole. When you feel that you know where you are aiming, try to put the peg into that hole without you or it touching the board and without making any adjustments if you notice you are off target as the peg gets close to the hole. If you miss start again and take as many tries as you need to get it in without contacting the board." I explain that this appears to be the simplest of tasks, but actually is quite difficult if done according to the instructions. I also try to make it clear that mistakes are an essential aspect of learning and improving. Here I am reminded of something mentioned earlier that Dr. Gregory Kitchener uses in his office and shared with me; "My job is to make this a safe place for you to make mistakes, your job is to make as many mistakes as necessary to complete the task I've laid out for you." This is important since we are often afraid to make mistakes. As children many of us had to deal with teachers who chided our mistakes and made us feel bad for having made them. This is absurd. Mistakes are essential for growth and development. The only caveat is that we do need to recognize and learn from our mistakes. But make them we must.

Eye movements

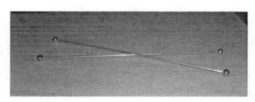

Figure 3.

Eye movements are probably the most basic visual skill. Accurate, consistent, effortless eye movements are critical in determining where things are, what they are, and then helping to guide our actions in response to that information. There are many possible ways to work on eye movements, but I cannot imagine anything better than a face-to-face approach. The eye movement procedure I do is derived from the work of Bruce Wolff, OD and the Behavioral Vision Project, which has been carrying on the legacy of Dr. Wolff.

Wolff wands (Figure 3) are the object of choice for several reasons. They are shiny and therefore attention-getting; the patient can fixate on their own small reflection in the ball. The ball presents a distinctive and excellent target to monitor focusing; and the ball is small enough not to get in the way of direct observation. Pursuits and saccades are done monocularly and then binocularly.

I move the ball in circles that move closer and farther from the person, going horizontally, vertically and diagonally. The movements are slow and smooth, typically moving between three and twenty-some inches from the face.

The person is seated on an adjustable-height stool with both feet flat on the floor or a footstool. They are instructed to sit up straight with the head straight with their hands placed palms-up on their knees. And finally they are instructed to keep their head still as they follow the ball wherever it goes. My job is to observe the person's ability to accurately, smoothly, and easily follow the target and to help keep them on target when their mind and eyes wander. How is the body posture as time goes on? Head posture? Is there excessive blinking? Are the two eyes similar in function? Do they work together properly?

Vectograms and Tranaglyphs

I talked about 3-D movies and eye teaming in the introduction. Doctors providing vision therapy have been using 3-D technology for over 50 years. The newer 3-D technology is quite advanced, but the principles are basically the same. Two very similar images are presented, one seen by the right eye and one by the left. We perceive the resulting imagery as three-dimensional when the brain is integrating all of this properly. Briefly, behavioral optometrists use 3-D glasses and images to evaluate and train eye teaming. We typically use 2 main types of 3-D: 1) Vectograms, which use polarized glasses and targets, and 2) Tranaglyphs, an older technology which uses red and green glasses with red and green targets. These targets can be manipulated to change where the image appears in space, that is, we can make it appear closer or farther.

These are just some examples of vision therapy procedures. There are many more and every doctor has their favorites. It is not so much the particular procedure that matters. It is the totality of the program and the thinking behind it that are important. These particular procedures are done by every person I work with if at all possible.

There is one more aspect of vision therapy that has only been mentioned briefly so far—LENSES. In my opinion, lenses are an extremely important part of any full-scope vision therapy program. It is important here to distinguish between the purpose of lenses used in the context of a vision therapy program and those typically received as the result of a standard eye exam. That is the subject of our next chapter.

Chapter Five

LENSES

The vast majority of practitioners who examine people's eyes look at lenses strictly as a way to eliminate obvious symptoms such as nearsightedness, farsightedness, and/or astigmatism, as well as improper eye alignment in some cases. These lenses are typically called *corrective* lenses, but they are more accurately considered *compensating* lenses since they merely compensate for some specific symptom and do not actually correct the underlying problem. I would expect corrective lenses to correct the problem, but they only mask it, often making the problem - and the symptom they were supposed to correct - worse over time. I prefer, whenever possible, to prescribe lenses that actually do help to correct visual problems. It seems that most eye care professionals are fairly nonchalant when it comes to prescribing lenses. If the patient can read the bottom line on the chart, or the eyes appear straight while wearing the lenses, chalk one up in the win column. That's just not good enough for most behavioral optometrists.

There are other ways to use lenses that began with the pioneering work of A. M. Skeffington, who, in the 1930s, began to understand the complexity, development, and plasticity of the human visual processing system. Skeffington realized that the strength of optometric care was not the treatment of an optical system but rather in treating the visually guided behavior and performance of each person. Most compensating lenses are prescribed on the basis of just one or two simple tests. This may provide some immediate relief of certain symptoms, but will not lead to any overall, long-term improvement and may actually have a negative influence on the overall visual process and its future development.

There are two main varieties of lenses that are used to manipulate light. The first device is what we all know of as a lens. The primary effect of a lens is changing the focus of light. That is, it will cause light to focus in front of or behind where it would normally focus (depending on whether the lens is convex or concave) in the absence of a lens. The second type of lens is known as a prism. The primary function of a prism is to bend light. Light will be deflected from its normal straight-ahead path when it passes through a prism, which makes the object (and everything else seen through the prism) appear shifted from its actual position. It is also important to know that a lens has some prismatic effects, and a prism has some lens-like effects, especially when you take into account how a person interacts with the lens. As I learned early on in my optometric career from my mentor and friend, Dr. Robert Kraskin, the important thing is not so much what a lens does, but what a person does in response to the lens. This is a cornerstone of the behavioral optometric philosophy.

It is a fairly simple matter of physics and optics to predict what will happen in the laboratory with light, lenses, and prisms. It is a much different story when there is a person involved. Each person has a somewhat unique response when looking through a lens or prism. While there are some consistencies in people's responses to particular lenses and prisms, there are almost always at least subtle differences from one individual to the next. Sometimes the responses can be quite different from what is expected. These differences can be critical in understanding an individual's level of visual development and sophistication, and in determining how a person will be able to benefit from the lenses or prisms.

A thorough visual evaluation is critical in determining the nature of the condition and the subsequent treatment of developmental/ functional visual disorders. Behavioral optometrists provide state-of-the-art care for strabismus.

As a result of Skeffington's ideas, the discipline of behavioral optometry was fortunate to avail itself of what may be the most potent tool for the safe, judicious, and gentle yet powerful manipulation of visual performance. The ability to utilize lenses for the enhancement of visual performance or the prevention of visual problems became a viable alternative with consistent results in a wide variety of applications. Sadly, it is a minority of practitioners who have invested the time to explore the possibilities of using lenses more dynamically and creatively. Those who have avoided expanding their philosophy often refuse to accept that these possibilities exist. Based on my clinical experience, the ability to enhance visual performance through the use of therapeutic lenses is too important a concept to remain unused by the vast majority of those prescribing lenses on a daily basis. The accurate diagnosis, based on a thorough functionally and developmentally oriented visual evaluation, is critical in determining the subsequent treatment of developmental/functional visual disorders through the use of therapeutic lenses and vision therapy. Behavioral optometry provides a state-of-the-art approach that should be as much a part of "standard of care" as all the latest medical, mechanical, and technological advances.

How do therapeutic lenses differ from other lenses? The lenses themselves are essentially the same. After all, as stated earlier, a lens does what a lens does. It is up to the doctor to determine the lenses that are most likely to lead to changes in visual development and therefore to the desired outcome. The nature of the evaluation process leading up to the actual prescription, the philosophy behind the recommendations for wearing the lenses, and the intention behind the way the lenses are prescribed and utilized determine the difference in the way the lenses influence visual development and performance. Vision therapy is usually necessary to optimize the person's ability to get the most out of their lenses, especially in cases of strabismus.

Similarly, the right lenses can often enhance the person's ability to get the most out of vision therapy. They simply go hand-in-hand in my experience. Prisms can also be used in a more therapeutic way. Prisms can be prescribed that will stimulate the brain to discover new patterns of visual performance. However, these kinds of prisms are rarely, if ever, utilized by any doctors other than behavioral optometrists. These are called *yoked prisms*, which are not used to compensate for some cosmetic deviation, but instead are used to stimulate positive changes in the brain. Yoked prisms (the description of which is not necessary for our purposes) help to bring about changes in overall visual behavior, which in turn leads to improvement that will be long lasting. The simple application of appropriate lenses and/or therapeutic prisms can go a long way towards reducing both the functional problem and the accompanying symptoms. It should be the goal of any therapeutic approach to improve the overall visual process and its development in all cases of visual difficulty.

This is a very important issue. A compensating lens is one that is designed to take over some function that is beyond the capability of the individual at that time. The use of compensating lenses usually arises from the opinion that the condition is an irreversible one, in fact one that is likely to worsen over time. It will continue to worsen until, for some inexplicable reason, it becomes stable, though not likely better. Compensating lenses do nothing to address the possible *cause* of the problem, and as a result, they do not provide any means of improving the underlying condition. The use of compensating lenses is a passive response to what is considered to be a passive problem. The standard eye exam has nothing in the diagnostic method and nothing in the subsequent treatment that even begins to address the dynamic and developmental nature of most visual problems.

I can't overemphasize the idea that it is not what a lens does, but what a person does in response to the lens that is important. The real importance of the ability to affect positive changes with lenses is the fact that the visual process is in many ways the most important interface between a person and his environment. We must have a highly accurate and flexible means of interpreting our world in order to achieve the highest level of performance, with maximum comfort and efficiency and a minimum of effort, if we are to hold our own in a fast paced, visually demanding, and visually stressful culture. When the brain is unable to integrate the two eyes properly it interferes with the accurate interpretation of our world. Vision therapy is a successful treatment option in the vast majority of these situations and therapeutic lenses are typically a crucial aspect of this process.

The ability to compensate for the variety of visual conditions mentioned earlier is unquestionably of benefit within our culture. People need to be able to see clearly at all distances under a variety of conditions with unhesitating flexibility and accuracy. They also need to be able to use both eyes together efficiently and comfortably. It is not too difficult to provide compensating lenses that do what they are intended to do. However, the use of compensating lenses to treat symptoms is an incomplete means of dealing with most visual problems. There are ways to assess and address the visual developmental deficiencies at the root of most visual problems. These techniques are the bread-and-butter of behavioral optometric practice. People must become better informed and demand a higher level of care. There is nothing exotic or difficult about the concepts utilized by behavioral optometrists. There is considerable scientific evidence that behavioral optometry is on the right track and on the cutting edge of managing functional and developmental difficulties of the visual process. The concepts utilized by behavioral optometrists do, however, require at least a little curiosity and a drive to provide more elaborate style of care for people in need.

The art of prescribing lenses has changed very little over the years for the majority of those providing standard eye care. The one glaring exception to this began, as mentioned earlier, with the thinking of Skeffington and others and later those who followed their lead. These pioneers were interested not only in prescribing the best possible compensating lenses but came to understand that lenses (and vision therapy) could also be used to prevent functional vision problems, to protect the visual system from stress and strain, and to improve or remediate visual problems that were already present whether causing obvious symptoms or not.

Behavioral optometry has maintained and improved upon the philosophy of dynamic and strategic lens prescribing throughout the years. The use of bifocals or reading lenses in children is one example. The constant use of the visual process within arm's reach is a common and frequent source of strain on the system. The problem is compounded even further when near work is done with the addition of stress to perform at a certain level. The judicious use of anti-stress reading lenses for those whose visual systems have begun to show the signs of compromise can be instrumental in preventing a more serious long-term breakdown in visual performance, as well as providing some structure upon which the visual process can build as it continues to develop.

Although our visual systems were not designed for the type of activities that we must do to "survive" in our culture, some of us seem quite able to handle the load. A significant percentage of us, however, are unable to maintain an adequate level of performance without significant stress on the visual system. This stress will often, sometimes sooner and sometimes later, cause adverse reactions including refractive changes (particularly nearsightedness and astigmatism), breakdown of binocular (eye teaming) integration, focusing anomalies, task avoidance, etc. Along with many of these functional problems, there can often be more obvious signs such as headaches, dry eyes, eye discomfort, fatigue, reduced efficiency, etc.

Optometric findings reveal the outward signs of how a person has adapted and compensated, mostly subconsciously, for visual inefficiencies in carrying out everyday tasks.

The findings of a visual evaluation and the diagnosis that emerges from the evaluation only describes where the visual system is at that moment in time. The findings provide a snapshot of the manner in which that person responded to visual challenges that were not being optimally handled at the time. The diagnosis merely provides a label and a definition of the visual condition at that time, not what caused it. The doctor must rely on his or her experience and skill and use the information gleaned from the evaluation to understand what is beneath the surface, to understand the original difficulties leading to the adaptations seen at the present time. These are the primary issues that need to be addressed during the treatment process.

Most undesirable visual adaptations and consequent findings result from some inability to handle the load placed on the visual system by some task or demand that is persistent over time. Adaptations are often indispensable (especially when the visual process has not developed to the expected degree) in order to come to terms with the demand of the task with the least amount of effort or discomfort.

It is possible to prevent the onset, slow down, or even reverse the progression of nearsightedness, farsightedness, and astigmatism. Lenses used in a dynamic, therapeutic way, usually in conjunction with vision therapy, can also help prevent or remediate strabismus. In all cases, it is a matter of looking at these conditions as results of delays or gaps in visual development and some fundamental difficulty with visual processing. The most powerful tool for bringing about positive changes in visual processing is a pair of low powered convex (plus) lenses. The use of appropriate plus lenses, with a therapeutic intention, with or without the benefit of vision therapy, can go a long way towards normalizing eye teaming, focusing, visual spatial perception, and peripheral visual awareness. Therapeutic lenses differ from compensating lenses in many ways. Therapeutic lenses are not intended to provide immediate improvement in acuity at any distance. They are not designed to take over some function of the optical system. Therapeutic lenses serve to enhance overall visual function by providing new instructions to the brain and will lead to positive changes over time. Therapeutic lenses are derived from a thorough evaluation of the entire visual process, not just the eye chart across the room.

Lenses are a type of medicine even though they are not taken internally. They can promote changes in behavior or affect the way one feels. Appropriate therapeutic lenses can promote positive changes in school performance and behavior as well as work performance. These lenses can also bring about changes in a person's level of comfort by eliminating eyestrain, eye pain, or headaches. Lenses change the incoming information, signals, and feedback to the brain. Therapeutic lenses do so in a purposeful way. And while there is no way to predict the exact way any particular brain will respond, an experienced behavioral optometrist can help steer the process in the right direction.

While in some cases compensating lenses can be seen to provide some of these same benefits, these changes are typically seen only when the lenses are being worn. This is not unlike some types of internally taken medications. They are effective only during an active phase, and when this phase elapses, the symptoms return and more medication is required to stop the symptoms. Therapeutic lenses will promote more long lasting changes. In fact, it is generally the case that such changes will become permanent, since the action of therapeutic lenses is to stimulate internalized changes in behavior and performance.

Another similarity between compensating lenses and standard medications is the likelihood of unwanted side effects. Although most medications will provide the desired changes while they are active, everything comes at some cost. In the case of most medications, that cost is unwanted and undesirable side effects. An analogous lens example would be the lenses used for nearsightedness. These lenses certainly cause a nearsighted person to see clearly at further distances, but they cause many unwanted side effects. Distance lenses cause the visual system to undergo increased strain if they are worn for close work, which is often the case. This frequently causes the person to become even more nearsighted and often leads to more complex visual disturbances such as eye teaming, focusing, and eye movement dysfunction.

Another example of unwanted side effects from lenses comes from the kind of prism typically prescribed for people with eye turns. In some cases, but not all, these prisms will cause the eyes to appear aligned while they are being worn. Once they are removed, their benefits disappear. In addition, they cause other complications in overall, long-term visual performance and comfort. There is a very good example of this in Chapter Eight: *How Do You Solve a Problem Like Maria?*

The more holistic approach to lenses taken by many behavioral optometrists stimulates the brain in ways that promote new and better visual habits and development. This approach provides options for perceiving and responding to the environment. Subconsciously, we are constantly searching for the path of least resistance and most effectiveness. It is difficult to achieve this if we do not have options from which to choose. Without a broader context, we can only know what is available to us. We have more power to select what suits us when there are choices available to us these days thanks to the vast amount of information available to us via the internet. I hope this book will get you thinking, asking questions, and searching for the information you need and deserve..

Another way to describe the intentions and effects of lenses is that compensating lenses attempt to deal with what has already happened and nothing more. Therapeutic lenses attempt to address what has already happened while at the same time providing a solid foundation for the continued development and improvement of the visual process.

Chapter Six

EYE MUSCLE SURGERY

Eye muscle surgery, also known as strabismus surgery, is the second most frequently performed ophthalmologic procedure after cataract surgery.[1,2] I learned from someone who had several eye muscle surgeries as a young child and had subsequently done considerable research on the subject, that a doctor can do as many as 14 of these procedures in a single day. According to one author, one of the great values of this procedure is its relatively low cost compared to other surgical procedures. "That strabismus surgery is compensated at a higher rate, than for example, cataract surgery, suggests that strabismus surgery is an excellent value."[1] It is difficult to figure out exactly what that means except that if you're in the mood for surgery and don't have a lot of money, this is the procedure for you. Otherwise, you had best be very wary.

It is well accepted by those who perform strabismus surgery that when performing the exact same procedure on two individuals, one should *not* expect identical results.[9-11,13,14] A search of the literature showed that the standard for a successful surgical outcome includes the presence of a fairly significant turning of the eye(s) in either direction (in or out) as measured at four weeks to six months postoperatively.[2,9,10,15,16] It makes sense that this kind of outcome is acceptable to surgeons because they continue to see the visual process as simply a collection of parts that enables us to see clearly. The only parts with which they are concerned are the eyeballs and their muscles, and in some cases some nerves that may be involved. As has been pointed out earlier, the visual process is mainly a brain process, not an eyeball/eye muscle phenomenon.

Just to be clear, let's say your child's eye was turning in on a constant basis. Strabismus surgery is performed and the eyes look straight immediately after the procedure. Sometime later, could be days or weeks, months or years, the eyes are no longer straight. It is entirely possible that the eye that used to turn inward is turning out instead. According to the medical standards, it does not matter which direction the eye is inappropriately pointing, as long as the degree of the turn is within a certain (arbitrary) amount. As it turns out, the brain has a much more difficult time integrating the changes if the eye is turning the opposite way post-surgically from what it did prior to surgery. This scenario, which is not at all uncommon, presents a monumental obstacle to developing better eye teaming, visual efficiency, and visual comfort, and of course keeping the eyes straight.

Some authors have begun to realize that the one to six month follow-up period is inadequate due to the frequency of deterioration of ocular alignment over time,[2] and that these patients should be reevaluated after four years to get a more accurate picture of the true results of these procedures.[15,17] As many doctors working towards functional improvement know, even four years is probably insufficient. If there is any meaningful cut-off time for the staying power of eye muscle surgery, it would be no less than five years.

The prevalence of reoperations is so great that most of the literature and numerous websites featuring strabismus FAQs mention the need for multiple surgeries very matter of factly,[1,8-11] and a great number of articles had the word "reoperation" in the title. Apparently it is not really considered a negative factor if an individual should need multiple procedures.[10,11,17] "Looked at another way, if the eyes are straight at any time after (eye muscle) surgery, the surgery itself has been effective. Moreover, (eye muscle) surgery that is done carefully can be repeated effectively and without compromise to the patient."[1] I find it stunning that surgeons can be satisfied with the eyes being straight "*at* any time" after surgery. Apparently they are not concerned with how long the eyes remain straight, just that they look straight for even a moment. I can't say for sure that this was the exact meaning of the statement, but it would take some effort to imagine another interpretation.

I was also taken aback at the ease with which they seem ready to do surgery all over again, however many times it takes, completely ignoring the permanent damage to the muscle(s) caused by each procedure. I know I have made the point repeatedly that the visual process is one that mostly occurs in the brain, but that does not negate the need for healthy, fully functioning eye muscles, able to carry out the instructions from the brain effortlessly, instantaneously, and accurately. None of this is ever quite the same once an eye muscle has been damaged - surgically or otherwise. Vision therapy after eye muscle surgery can often be very successful, but the permanent and substantial restriction of normal muscle function that results from the scar tissue and the destruction of the special fibers telling the brain where the eye is pointing, makes everything more difficult.

Proof of the prevalence of the surgical way of thinking is demonstrated by one of the most significant advances in these procedures, the principles of which "have remained essentially unchanged since the mid-19th century, when this surgery was first done"[1] - adjustable sutures.[9,18] This technique so blatantly admits the uncertainty surrounding eye muscle surgery as to be beyond the obvious, verging on the absurd. This procedure provides for an adjustment to be made a day or so after the surgery has been "completed," if it is felt that some fine tuning is in order. One other innovation which appeared around the same time (the late 1970s) was botulinum toxin injection, used to create a partial paralysis of the eye muscle(s).[18] This requires an injection of the toxin into the particular muscle or muscles that supposedly need weakening.

I want to go back briefly to a quote from above. "Looked at another way, if the eyes are straight at any time after (eye muscle) surgery, the surgery itself has been effective."[1] I interpret this statement to mean that if the eyes look straight for even a brief moment at any time after the procedure, this is deemed successful strabismus surgery. Obviously strabismus surgery is not an easy procedure. One reason it is not easy is that the magnitude of the eye turn often varies from moment to moment and may further vary depending on the particular task in which the person is engaged. Also, some cases of strabismus are intermittent to begin with. This means that the eye turn only happens periodically, and yet even these cases are considered fair game for strabismus surgery by many surgeons. I cannot fathom the thought process leading to the conclusion that a permanent structural change would be a good way to treat an intermittent problem that is clearly not physical in nature. It is also common for strabismus to alternate, that is, sometimes one eye is turning inappropriately, sometimes the other. The decision of which eye to operate on under these conditions wasn't clear from my research. Another way to think about this is that most vision difficulties are software issues, not bad hardware. You can fix a software problem without replacing critical parts of your computer.

As I write this, I have over 25 years of personal experience working with people of all ages to eliminate or at least better manage their strabismus. This does not include the year I spent as a vision therapy patient during my first year in optometry school. This does include working with: my brother many years after having wrongly assumed his strabismus surgery had fixed everything, my father who began having intermittent double vision in his 70s and my daughter (beginning at the age of 5), for whom I was able to prevent the need for eye muscle surgery. More about my brother and daughter in the final chapter. I have worked with children whose parents wanted to avoid surgery, and in most cases I have been able to help these children - as young as 2 years of age - learn how to keep their eyes straight and, more important, working together.

These changes are permanent in most cases. It was only a matter of tuning things up a little in the small percentage of people who did not maintain 100% of their improvement permanently. In fact, the most common scenario I see is that once a person has completed their vision therapy program, their visual abilities continue to improve on their own as time goes on. This happens because the changes triggered by vision therapy are changes in the brain, and those changes ultimately become part of the brain's default behavior, allowing the visual process to develop atop a more stable and extensive foundation from that time forward.

I can tell you without hesitation that it is much harder to help someone who has had strabismus surgery than someone who has not, in most cases. Part of this is simply the reduced flexibility of the eye muscles after surgery, and some is the significant confusion the brain must deal with when an eye muscle has been surgically altered. Another problem is the previously mentioned, and not at all uncommon, condition where an eye that turned toward the nose prior to surgery begins to turn away from the nose after surgery. As mentioned, this presents almost insurmountable difficulty for the brain when there is no vision therapy involved. There is also the fairly common problem of leaving the eyes with a vertical misalignment after surgery. This is also very difficult for the brain to manage effectively, even with vision therapy. Surgeons will typically offer surgery to correct this.

Any surgery is risky, especially when it involves general anesthesia, as does eye muscle surgery. However, the follow-up treatment is extremely important. It seems only a matter of common sense that any damage to a functional body part should be followed by a functionally oriented therapeutic regimen. This is true whether the damage is caused by surgery or by trauma. If a muscle is strained or sprained, it is first rested and then exercised. The protocol is the same if a muscle is damaged and repaired. Particularly if we are working under the assumption that eye muscles are at fault in the majority of strabismus cases,[8] which has absolutely no basis in fact, the almost total lack of active follow-up care defies logic. It is well understood and accepted that there is more to effective eye teaming than mere alignment of the eyes. In fact, comfortable and effective eye alignment depends on accurate and effortless brain activity, not the other way around. It is the brain that tells the eyes where to point and how to communicate and integrate with each other. Why then is there no attempt made by surgeons to maximize the possibility of achieving sophisticated, coordinated binocular vision?

Surgery to straighten the eyes is based on the assumption that realigning the eyes so they will appear straight to an outside observer will fix everything. I have examined hundreds of people who would be candidates for eye muscle surgery. More and more parents tell me the surgeon said there was nothing wrong with their child's eye muscles, but surgery on the healthy muscle(s) is the only way to straighten the eyes. These parents were completely bewildered by this pronouncement, as am I–though this seems like a step in the right direction for the surgeons to acknowledge this. Most surgeons still believe that most poorly aligned eyes are due to faulty muscles as far as I can tell. Again, even if this was true, the overall thinking is still problematic due to the lack of accounting for the complexity of the visual process.

There are standard testing procedures which assess the structural and functional integrity of all the eye muscles. I routinely perform these tests on every patient in my office, including people who have cosmetically misaligned eyes. I have seen very few people with damaged eye muscles without having had eye muscle surgery. Yet many people who exhibit properly functioning eye muscles are still told by surgeons that strabismus surgery is the only treatment to get the eyes to be straight.

Many children (and adults) have eye turns that are not only in-termittent, but they also have what is called alternating strabismus, which means that sometimes one eye wanders off target, sometimes the other. Again, I must claim ignorance as to how a surgical pro-cedure, which is permanent and affects every action carried out by the muscle that was operated on, would be a good idea for a prob-lem that only occurs under certain conditions. Let's say you live in Pennsylvania and it's the middle of winter, you're visiting the doctor wearing shorts and a T-shirt and you explain that you are finding it hard to keep warm. Clearly the problem here is that you are inappropriately dressed considering the weather and the fact that you feel cold. The doctor suggests you wear insulated pants and a heavy parka...and not just during the winter, but all-year round. This would very likely solve the problem of feeling chilled during the winter, but might cause some problems come spring and sum-mer. At least you might come to your senses and realize there is a problem with this strategy and wake up one August morning and take off the winter wear. Surgery of course, is not something you can decide to ignore once it's been completed.

Common wisdom holds that after strabismus surgery, the af-fected muscle permanently loses a significant amount of its flex-ibility. Imagine how this adds up with multiple procedures. There is no question that the muscle can never regain its former ability after damage by surgery though the exact amount may be unknown. Most important may be the specialized fibers, described previously, located in the part of the muscle that is cut, where the muscle attaches to the eyeball. These particular fibers relay important information to the rest of the brain relating the precise position of that muscle and therefore the eye. The brain needs this crucial information to fine tune the signals it sends to the eyes and body in order to enable us to carry out every action in the most effective, efficient way possible. This is probably a big reason why so many people have so little success in using their two eyes the way they were meant to be used after eye muscle surgery. Vision therapy is an excellent way to overcome these difficulties instead of, or even after, strabismus surgery.

The cause of eye teaming problems would seem to be an important issue in determining a course of treatment. In my search of the literature, the cause is typically mentioned only when describing those cases excluded from a retrospective study, which looks at patient files from previous surgeries. The causes were also mentioned when describing the fact that the origins of eye teaming problems are still a point of disagreement, as has been the case since the beginning of the debate over a hundred years ago. One side in this discussion states that the brain's inability to keep the eyes in proper alignment is the main cause, and the other states that the eye muscles are unable to coordinate properly.[18,19] There also continues to be complete disagreement on when to perform eye muscle surgeries.[17,20] Some suggest that there is a significant difference in results and surgical effects among developmentally delayed children, including those with cerebral palsy, hydrocephalus, seizure disorder, and Down Syndrome.[21] If there are problems with predicting the outcome of these procedures in normal children, and there most certainly are, it seems that those with more complex needs present an even greater uncertainty, at least according to the medical literature.

Another issue that I did not see mentioned in any of the articles I reviewed was the effect such surgeries have on an individual's performance, behavior, and psyche. The closest thing I saw was mention of changes in spatial perception post-operatively, that is, the ability to accurately perceive distances based on visual input: eye teaming/depth perception. Eye teaming is of critical importance for behavioral optometrists in determining the quality of visual development and function. Eye teaming also tends to be important to the person using the eyes and should be at least a consideration going in to eye muscle surgery. It typically is not.

I have witnessed various effects that were directly attributable to surgery and many that were very likely the result of surgery over the years. One patient spent years battling with her surgeon over her complaints of severe discomfort whenever trying to use her eyes; she was told that it was all in her head, to stop thinking about it so much, and was summarily dismissed as a nuisance. Her visual discomfort and functional problems were clearly real as evidenced by my initial evaluation and subsequent work with her in vision therapy. Another patient came into my office with a severe eye and head twitch, severe in both magnitude and frequency. I was amazed that he had not sustained a neck injury. A 6 year old I examined less than a year after having eye muscle surgery reported that her eyes "feel like they're melting."

Practitioners providing vision therapy are constantly required to defend that method of treatment based on medical necessity. Behavioral optometrists would rarely consider cosmetic appearance as the primary reason for therapy, and never as the primary goal. One article cited "Compromised Appearance (Poor Self Image)" under the heading "Indications" for surgery; this was listed along with double vision and inability of the eye muscles of the two eyes to coordinate, as well as abnormal head posture and nystagmus (constant or frequent shaking of the eyes).[1] The inclusion of cosmetic appearance as an indication of the need for surgery was obviously an attempt to classify a cosmetic problem as a medical condition, warranting medical/surgical intervention. Cosmetic surgery is rarely covered by insurance and I imagine the number of people opting for eye muscle surgery would be much smaller if it was not covered by medical insurance. I wish the surgeons would focus more on the importance of visual development and function and make those issues the primary reasons for attempting to straighten the eyes. Then we could all work together as a team to provide the highest level of care and improvement for every patient.

I was also surprised to learn that as new procedures are developed, they are tried out on humans as seemingly routine events.[22] Of course, from my perspective, most strabismus surgery seems fairly experimental, and my search of the medical literature has done nothing but reinforce this perception. There are also variations on how eye muscle surgery is carried out. Some doctors will shorten one muscle, some will lengthen that muscle's partner. Some will operate on both at the same time. There seemed to be no set protocol and the results were generally determined to be just fine by medical standards. As discussed previously, behavioral optometrists have very demanding standards by which they determine how successful vision therapy has been. These standards are all about the quality of eye teaming and spatial/depth perception, focusing and eye movements and the quality of life. Behavioral optometrists are not satisfied with merely having the eyes appear straight for some brief period of time.

There continues to be frequent criticism from the medical community that the concepts and methods of behavioral optometry are not grounded in scientific proof. This is completely untrue. I grew tired of hearing these unjustified claims, which led me to investigate the scientific basis of strabismus surgery. That's what inspired me to write this book. To this end I read nearly 100 articles from various medical journals. Most were written by surgeons, some of whom also taught surgical techniques for strabismus surgery. Imagine my surprise in finding absolutely no scientific support, let alone proof, for routinely performing irreversible surgical procedures on people's eye muscles, most of which are perfectly healthy according to time-honored testing methods.

The causes of strabismus are still poorly understood; the medical procedures have an effectiveness that varies wildly. There is no way to predict the amount of change in eye alignment per amount of surgery. So far, the best answer to this problem is adjustable sutures, a procedure that is now skewing the data since these adjustments are not considered re-operations. There is no guarantee, nor any way of predicting, whether or not the immediate postoperative realignment of the eyes will remain intact or for what length of time. There is little data on the effects these procedures have on how the eyes will work as a team; the little information there is in this regard is as inconclusive as the information on all the other aspects of strabismus surgery. Actually, calling this information inconclusive is a little unfair. There is a fairly consistent pattern to all this information. The concepts, procedures, and results of strabismus surgery in general are extremely weak from the ground up.

Optometric vision therapy continues to achieve better results for many people who are otherwise considered to be good candidates for surgery, with none of the drawbacks of surgical intervention. Vision therapy also continues to be of tremendous value to people of all ages who have already had eye muscle surgery and are at some point, for one reason or another, dealing with any of a number of functional deficits and/or complaints of reduced comfort. Many of these people are struggling with headaches, eye fatigue and discomfort, double vision, reduced quality of and endurance for visual performance, and often reduced quality of life. When they go to the surgeon with these complaints all they are offered is more surgery. I have interviewed dozens of people who had eye muscle surgery though were not my patients. They all seem to avoid various activities that they would like to be doing, not realizing that visual discomfort was the reason for avoiding them. Vision therapy would very likely help these people enjoy doing these things again. When they go to the surgeon with these complaints all they are offered is more surgery. The woman I saw who had 10 eye muscle surgeries could barely move that eye in any direction.

One of the most shocking revelations I unearthed during my research was the fact that it has been found that there is no significant difference in the outcomes of surgeries performed by specialists as compared to those performed by generalists.[2] This means that those surgeons who perform these procedures on a routine basis were getting results no different from surgeons who only performed these procedures occasionally. While this finding was quite unnerving to me, the authors found it to be "reassuring." I would have hoped that a surgeon who performed strabismus surgery on a regular basis would have much better outcomes than one who only did these surgeries on rare occasions, but this has not been the case. Apparently experience does count for something in many other surgical procedures. "In fact, a recent landmark research study published in the *New England Journal of Medicine* solidified what most doctors and nurses already knew. Using national data, a leading health-services research group from the University of Michigan found that surgical death rates are directly related to a surgeon's experience with that particular operation. The researchers found the same relationship for many types of surgical procedures."[23]

One very good thing I can say about strabismus surgery is that the mortality rate has gone way down over the years. It is now a rare occurrence. This is mostly due to advances in anesthesia, which had been implicated in a significant number of deaths during strabismus surgery in the past.

Chapter Seven

WHAT TO LOOK FOR

Some visual problems are fairly obvious to a familiar observer, like a family member or teacher. Others are very subtle and will only be picked up by a trained observer during the course of the kind of thorough developmental visual evaluation performed by a behavioral optometrist. There may be obvious symptoms or functional deficits that cry out for special care, or there may be difficulties that are thought to be completely unrelated to what you think of as vision—what I have been calling the visual process. Sorting through all of this can be especially tricky when we are told by an expert eye care professional that the eyes are perfectly healthy, can see clearly, and therefore cannot be the cause of any problems. I see this in my office on a regular basis. Many people I work with have been seen previously (and sometimes recently) by other very competent practitioners only to be told that their eyes are healthy and can see 20/20 and therefore their complaints are unrelated to the visual process. The only problem is that they are not visually comfortable or are not performing at the level they would expect. My evaluation typically uncovers the visual issues causing the complaints.

Typical complaints of people seeking my help include: frequent headaches, eye fatigue, general fatigue, inability to work at the computer or read for adequate periods of time, eye pain or discomfort, etc. The typical eye exam cannot explain the cause of these problems and therefore leads to the conclusion that the eyes are not at fault. In fact, this conclusion is fairly accurate - it is just not complete. The eyes are not at fault. It is the breakdown of the visual processing apparatus of the brain that causes many complaints and many cases of strabismus. This, in turn, leads to reduced visual efficiency, which then leads to reduced performance and/or physical discomfort.

If a person is observed to have an eye that tends to turn in or out at times, it would seem fairly obvious that something is not right. We have all seen enough people to know when someone's eyes look straight and appear to be working together. This is a pretty straight-forward situation. However, most strabismus, except in newborns or infants, started out as something less obvious. It usually takes a certain amount of time dealing with the problem before the eyes appear obviously misaligned. Once this occurs, the problem is pretty far along and will be more complicated to manage. It is important to know some of the earlier signs of visual problems. This may help in recognizing problems before they get even more complicated and difficult to manage.

Every child exhibiting developmental delays, including those either on or suspected of being on the autism spectrum, should be evaluated for delays in visual development. A child who displays difficulty making and/or sustaining eye contact should raise suspicions of visual difficulty as well. Any doubts regarding performance in reading, writing, or general coordination warrant a more thorough assessment of visual development and function. A child who tends to get very close to see things, or who seems to squint frequently should be properly evaluated, and not just for acuity. No harm can come from having a child evaluated by a behavioral optometrist. However, many conditions that are readily treated with proper lenses and/or vision therapy are likely to go undetected without the thorough visual evaluation done by behavioral optometrists.

In the case of a newborn or very young child, who has not yet begun to face the kinds of visual demands that can lead to problematic adaptations, there may be nothing other than the appearance of an eye that seems out of alignment with its partner. Most parents will not want to wait very long before seeking professional guidance in these cases. I suspect that most people still believe that a pediatric ophthalmologist should be the first choice. It's not a bad idea as far as making sure that there are no complicating circumstances, and ophthalmologists are generally very good at examining the physical structures of and around the eyes. However, once physical damage or some underlying disease process is ruled out, it is prudent to seek the advice of a behavioral optometrist. Only behavioral optometrists are equipped to assess the developmental and functional issues involved in evaluating and treating an eye turn within the framework of the total visual process, and this is something you really want to incorporate into your decision-making process. I hope I have convincingly spelled out the reasons for this.

In closing, I would just say that everyone wants the best, especially for their children. I am sure that every doctor is attempting to provide what he or she thinks is the best treatment for each person seeking their help. I embarked on this project simply to learn more about strabismus surgery and to share what I had learned, especially with parents anxiously searching for answers to some very specific questions such as: Why are my child's eyes not working together? How can I get that one eye to aim where it's supposed to? Is there more than one way to fix the problem? I hope this book will help you to do more thorough research in trying to answer these questions for yourself, because any "expert" you ask, myself included, is likely to give you an answer that is filtered by their specific area of expertise. Though my goal is always to be as objective as possible, I know that because of my personal and professional experiences, my answers to these questions have a particular bias.

There have been occasions where I felt that eye muscle surgery was indicated as part of the overall treatment, but the surgery was only part of the process, which absolutely included vision therapy and therapeutic lenses. It is up to you to sort through all the available information and choose what makes the most sense to you. I want to help make sure that you have as much information as possible before making a very important decision.

Please be sure to read the stories of people who have been helped with their strabismus thanks to behavioral optometry and vision therapy in the next chapter.

Chapter Eight

VISION THERAPY STORIES

This chapter includes stories of patients who have experienced significant difficulty with their vision. Some had eye muscle surgery, some were spared this ordeal thanks to pre-emptive vision therapy, and one had vision therapy before and after eye muscle surgery. This is a small sampling of people, all of whom were seen in my office. Some of these people had eye muscle surgery or multiple surgeries as children or teenagers. Maria began noticing double vision later in life; Barbara had surgery as part of her vision therapy program; Nova would have been a candidate for eye muscle surgery had it not been for vision therapy and developmental lenses. Behavioral optometrists the world over have similar stories to tell as do the thousands and thousands of people struggling with strabismus who have been helped by vision therapy. I hope these stories and this book will help you to make the best decision possible for your child or for you or someone you care about when considering how to proceed with the vision care you need.

Cynthia And The Big Blurry Spot

Cynthia gives a clear account of her visual history and her real life complaints at the time of her first visit and her experience with vision therapy:

I first came to Dr. Gallop with a constellation of complaints. The chief among them was a blurry spot in my vision that seemed to come and go. I had seen a neurologist with this complaint, but after checking the health of my eyes and my visual reflexes, he told me that there was nothing physically wrong and that I should just get used to it. Along with the blurry spot that had been plaguing me for a year or more, I was experiencing ever-increasing eye strain and accompanying headaches.* By the end of a day, I literally had to close my eyes to relieve the stress - taking off my glasses didn't seem to provide enough relief. I was fortunate enough to have an optometrist who knew about and believed in vision therapy and thought that it would be beneficial for me, particularly since I had under-

gone corrective [eye muscle] surgery for "lazy eye" when I was 10 years old. He referred me to Dr. Gallop.

I said earlier that I had several complaints - blurry vision, eye strain. I was also failing at being able to wear contact lenses. I had been able to use them successfully as a young teen, but at 35 I was less and less comfortable with them. I had even invested quite a bit of money in a pair that was specifically designed to correct astigmatism. By the time I saw Dr. Gallop, I was wearing my glasses almost exclusively - and wasn't happy about it.

After my very first visit, Dr. Gallop recommended that I put aside my glasses and begin to wear just one contact lens, which he prescribed. After only a day or so of adjustment, I was as happy as could be with the one lens. After several weeks had passed, my glasses (when I found myself using them) felt very uncomfortable. The eye strain disappeared. Now, almost a year later, it is impossible for me to tolerate my glasses for more than 15 minutes. In fact, I am convinced that I can see BETTER (not necessarily with more acuity, but better) without any correction than with those glasses.

The blurry spot that was bothering me seemed to fade away with the contacts for quite a while. Then, about two months ago, it came back. The doctor asked me to try wearing a pair of glasses that contain a mild prism and this does the trick. The more often I wear the glasses (just for short stretches) the less often the spots appear. Our next step will be to put these lenses into a pair of glasses of my own that I can more comfortably wear when I need them.

These results are those that I wanted to accomplish. Based on the way I am performing certain exercises during our sessions today compared to 11 months ago, I can also see that I am able to accomplish visual tasks that were impossible before. Dr. Gallop knows what all of that means, I just know that my visual life is greatly - really amazingly - improved. There is no doubt in my mind that my weekly sessions with Dr. Gallop are the cause for this change.

* The blurry spot referred to by Cynthia is commonly known as a "floater." I will not go into medical detail here, but floaters are quite common. This one, unfortunately, was often right in Cynthia's line of sight which is why it was so bothersome. The vision therapy and lenses helped Cynthia focus less on the floater and to expand her peripheral awareness, which also helped change the floater from the most obvious thing in her visual field to something more like background noise.

How Do You Solve A Problem Like Maria?

Maria came to me because of continuing problems with double vision. She first noticed the problem 15 years prior to our first meeting. She was first prescribed compensating prisms at the age of 76. Following two cataract surgeries, one month apart, at the age of 78, her double vision became much more noticeable and therefore problematic because the second image was much clearer. Double vision is often treated by putting prism lenses in front of the eyes. Doctors usually refer to these as 'corrective' prisms, but they don't actually correct anything. They essentially trick the brain into acting as if the eyes were properly aligned. That is why I refer to this kind of prism as 'compensating' prism. There is a strong tendency for the brain to adapt to the prisms and this leads to a need for stronger prisms. The strength of the prisms that were added to Maria's glasses went from 9^ to 20^ over a 4½ year period. Without going into too much detail here, I will say that even 9 is a fairly large amount of prism in my opinion.

When the double vision began bothering her again, even with 20^ of base out prism already in place the other doctors told Maria that they couldn't prescribe stronger prisms and that surgery was the only possible solution. Not being a fan of allopathic medicine, surgery was not something Maria even wanted to consider. She takes no medications, eats very healthy home-cooked meals and has had minimal contact with doctors throughout her life. It took significant coaxing to get Maria to agree to cataract surgery. Three different surgeons told her that the only way to eliminate her double vision was eye muscle surgery. Maria balked, finding it quite odd that none of these doctors had anything other than surgery to suggest. She just couldn't believe that this could be true.

Maria found me after a lengthy search for something other than what she had been told was the only possible way to fix her problem. Her search brought her into contact with Dr. Sue Barry who told her there was most definitely something else to try. When Maria called my office and I answered the phone, and then all of her questions, she was ready to start vision therapy. Maria's goal was to get her eyes straight without wearing prisms and without any more double vision.

Maria was 85 years old when we first met. She is a very personable and energetic woman, and she was excited to try something other than surgery and the massive prisms that had been her only hope to this point. As it turns out, the prisms were doing quite a bit more than tricking the visual system into behaving as though the two eyes were aiming and working in an integrated and efficient manner. What the prisms were most definitely not doing was helping her brain to learn how to use the two eyes in the most effective, integrated way. In Maria's case, she was often unintentionally using only one eye at a time. Her brain learned how to ignore the right eye since her right eye was the one that crossed most often.

An important note: there are two ways that people avoid seeing double. The preferred way is for the two eyes to work in an efficient, integrated way. The other way, which comes into play when the previous method is not happening, is for the brain to ignore the input from one eye. This can lead to other not-so-desirable adaptations, but is much more tolerable than seeing double.

Maria knew that vision therapy was her treatment of choice by the time she contacted me. She strongly believed that surgery should only be a last resort. She was excited to try a more dynamic and interactive approach having already experienced what compensating prisms as stand-alone treatment provided. I agree with Maria that surgery should be a last resort. I think that compensating prisms should be a close second-to-last option. Vision therapy is the treatment of choice for almost all types of eye turns. Vision therapy is almost always necessary to help develop more efficient and effective ways of using the two eyes together, whether or not surgery (or compensating prisms) is determined to be a useful adjunct.

Maria started vision therapy the week after her initial evaluation. At that visit we determined that she could use her eyes in an integrated way, within arm's reach, with just over half the amount of prism she had been wearing. I had glasses made with the reduced prism by Maria's third vision therapy session. I had her keep her old prescription because I assumed this new prescription would be challenging. The plan was to have her wear the reduced prisms as much as possible with the intention of gradually reducing the amount of prism in the most comfortable yet timely and effective way possible.

One of the first things I do with almost every vision therapy patient is to change the prescription they were using when we first met - prism or otherwise. Most prescriptions are based solely on trying to give the person the best visual acuity (eyesight) possible or trying to cosmetically align the eyes. These compensating lenses are based on what has happened in the past. They are a doctor's response to the patient's adaptations to their visual issues; they do not address the causes.

Let me explain this a little again. Most doctors do not think about why or how a person came to have the visual condition that the patient is concerned about or that the doctor will ultimately diagnose. Similarly, most doctors do not appreciate that the condition seen on the surface is usually the result of a person's difficulty using their visual system in an effortless, efficient manner. Maria was compensating for visual inefficiencies over many years without knowing it, which is a very common situation. We adapt to our visual difficulties in some way in order to use the visual process as best we can, usually without the slightest clue that we are even doing anything. It is also common for the brain to tire of all the extra work it has been doing to hold things together. This is when symptoms emerge, seemingly out of nowhere, when in fact they have simply been kept hidden by our adaptations and our unconscious effort.

I want to provide therapy and lenses that will help a person develop new, more effective, less effortful patterns. In Maria's case I knew that her old prisms would be working against the changes in visual behavior that we were trying to encourage with vision therapy. She needed something that would allow her visual process to develop in a different direction. Maria reported being able to wear the reduced prism prescription for only one to two hours, three to four times a day for the first week. By the second week she reported wearing them almost full-time, only relying on her old glasses for brief, specific situations.

After six weeks with her new prescription and weekly vision therapy sessions Maria informed me that she noticed that she was seeing better at distance without lenses than with them. I found this surprising, but the eye chart verified what Maria was telling me. She was seeing almost one whole line better on the eye chart without any lenses, and considerably better than with her old glasses. This brings up something I believe is important, but is quite different than what most eye doctors believe or would ever consider: Optimal visual acuity should be thought of as a result of a well-functioning visual process. It is not a prerequisite to getting the system to work in a more balanced or symmetrical way. I have found that vision therapy often leads to improved distance acuity with reduced lens powers or no lenses at all. This is because the person becomes able to make better use of the available information as the visual process becomes more sophisticated and effective thanks to vision therapy and/or a more strategic, dynamic use of lenses.

Approximately three months into therapy, since Maria was wearing her reduced prism prescription most of the time, I prescribed even weaker prisms - now about one quarter the strength of what she had when we first met. This provided appropriate distance and near visual acuities, but was difficult to use consistently due to the reduced prisms. It took Maria seven more months to begin using this prescription on a fairly consistent basis. By this time she was rarely using her original prescription.

After a few more sessions Maria started saying that she was feeling more secure and steady when walking. She was more confident in her sense of where she was in space and more confident of what her feet were doing. Maria realized that prior to seeing me she had become gradually less and less able to navigate unfamiliar terrain as her prisms increased until, by the time we met, she generally needed to hold her husband's hand because of her growing uncertainty in unfamiliar surroundings, including the mall. We talked about this and discussed the fact that Maria had her peripheral awareness practically taken away by the prisms. The strong prisms she was wearing were literally collapsing Maria's world, and not just her visual world. The prisms she was wearing for her particular condition - eye(s) turning in - tend to shrink the usable peripheral vision a person has. This is especially true as the prisms are increased in strength. Prisms used to compensate for crossed eyes basically shrink the world in all dimensions so that the person doesn't need to uncross their eyes to function. Maria, despite the massive prisms in her glasses, still had crossed eyes when we first met - even with her glasses on.

When I first met Maria she was bubbly personality-wise, but she was quite hunched over and tentative in her movements. I admit to being a bit ageist on this count, but I just assumed that at the age of 85 she had simply lost the ability to stand up as straight as I imagine she used to do. It also seemed reasonable that her age was a contributing factor to her hesitant movements. On the morning of Maria's 21st VT session I immediately noticed something was very different when she came in. She was standing up almost perfectly straight. She has stayed that way for the six months since. Maria recently renewed her driver's license and remarked, "When I compared my old picture with the new one, I was surprised to see that I look younger in the new picture than the one from several years ago. People that know me are commenting that something about me looks very different, and better than even a year ago. One great thing is that my handbag doesn't keep sliding off my shoulder as it has been for many years."

Maria's husband shared the following in writing around this time:

"The physical change in my wife's posture is most extraordinary. As prism strength increased over the last three or four years so too was it accompanied by an increase in a forward stooping of her neck and shoulders. As the prism strength has been reduced she has resumed more of her normal upright posture. If this continues at the present rate, normal posture is within sight. This is remarkable on several levels and worthy of some serious research."

The negative change in Maria's posture was not mentioned at our initial meeting and it did not occur to me that her posture was anything but age related - I will not make that mistake again.

Clearly Maria's life had been drastically altered by the long-term, constant use of such strong prisms. While there may have been some benefit to the prisms, which is by no means certain, there was a significant down-side. Little by little Maria's movement, posture and quality of life were being restricted. It was a gradual process and so went unnoticed for the most part, until the weaker prisms and vision therapy allowed her to glimpse what had been and what could be again. Maria has been doing all the vision therapy procedures described in Chapter 4 along with various others.

I am still working with Maria at the time of this writing. Excellent progress has already occurred on all counts. We will continue trying to decrease the strength of her prisms while increasing the stability and flexibility of her visual system and regaining the quality of life her old prism glasses had taken away. There is not as yet a happy ending but the trip has been most enjoyable for Maria and myself and the improvement so far is very encouraging. We are both looking forward to her continued improvement.

Barbara's Strabismus Surgery and Vision Therapy

Barbara came to my office because she could never aim her two eyes at the same thing at the same time. She was Jamaican, in her mid-20s, here on a temporary visa working as an au pair. Barbara was not seeing double, she just wanted her eyes to be straight. I explained to her that the best way to achieve this was to teach her brain to get the two eyes working together. After the initial evaluation I explained that she could see 20/20 with each eye, had adequate focusing abilities with each and that each eye had normal eye movements and ranges of motion of all the eye muscles. During the evaluation of Barbara's eye movements her two eyes would move together when following a target, but only one eye would aim at the target at any given time. The other eye would appear to be looking far off to the side away from her nose.

There was nothing wrong with any of the eye muscles, but her brain just wasn't able to integrate the two eyes properly. Barbara was simply unable to point both eyes at the same thing at the same time. That is, when she looked at you with her right eye, the left eye was pointing way off toward her left ear; when she looked at you with her left eye, the right eye was pointing way off toward her right ear. We decided to try vision therapy first, see where that would take us and then consider surgery if need be.

After three months of weekly vision therapy sessions and no significant observable change in Barbara's ability to converge her eyes, we decided that Barbara should seek a surgical consultation. I referred her to a local ophthalmologist who was fairly new to the area. This doctor had paid a visit to my office to introduce himself when he came to town. He ended up spending a fair amount of time in my office and seemed quite surprised and interested as I described and demonstrated vision therapy. He apparently had never heard of behavioral optometry or vision therapy. We were each hoping to get patients referred from the other. I was searching for a surgeon with whom I could work to best serve my patients.

Barbara met with the surgeon and came back for her next vision therapy session quite concerned. "The other doctor told me he was going to operate on both eyes," she told me, seeming considerably distressed. "I don't want him to operate on both eyes," she continued. I promised to contact him and find out exactly what he had suggested and to inquire about his rationale for his recommended approach. I called the surgeon and expressed Barbara's anxiety. He assured me that operating on both eyes made no sense and that he would only operate on one eye. The next week I relayed this message to Barbara and we decided to take a break from vision therapy until after the surgery.

Several weeks later, after the surgery, Barbara returned to my office, once again in obvious anguish. She told me that the surgery had been done on both eyes and that one eye was constantly bothering her. Barbara said that one eye felt fine, but the other felt strange most of the time. It is possible that the emotional trauma of being misled caused her to focus her attention on the eye that was supposed to be left intact, but it's also possible that the post-surgical sensation in that eye was in fact different and annoying. Either way, there was no reversing the situation since surgery is permanent. As discussed earlier in the book, there is always at least some degree of permanent damage to any eye muscle that has been surgically altered.

There was nothing left to do but to continue vision therapy in the hope that, now that the eyes were better aligned, we would have an easier time getting the brain to learn how to get the two eyes functioning as a team. I will never forget the day that Barbara first experienced true depth perception. She was doing an eye teaming activity* that involved what is known as physiological diplopia. Diplopia means double vision. Physiological diplopia is normal, though we usually are able to ignore it when it happens and there is typically no need to have awareness of it under normal seeing conditions. I had stepped out of the room for a moment while Barbara was doing the activity. Suddenly I heard Barbara scream and as I looked over at her she was jumping up and down, delighted and somewhat shocked. She described what she was seeing as if she had seen something other-worldly. What she was describing was seeing in three dimensions. She had never seen anything like it as far as she could remember. There were some ups and downs after that, which is not uncommon, but for the most part Barbara was able to see in three dimensions from then on.

* The activity was similar to this: Hold a finger, pointing at the ceiling, about 10 inches away, directly in front of your nose with some other object across the room, also directly in front of your nose. When you look at your finger you should see two of the distant object, optimally one on either side of your finger. When you look at the distant object, you should see two of your finger, optimally one off to either side of your nose. Barbara was doing this with the distant object being a specially designed target that would appear 3-D when everything was just right. The only way to see the 3-D image is to have both eyes (and the brain of course) working properly together. If you are not seeing what I have described, it's probably time to find a behavioral optometrist near you :-)

Neal Goes 3-D

Neal is my younger brother. He always struggled in school, especially with reading. He is almost as nearsighted as I am–which is quite a bit. His other visual issues were more severe than mine though they were never properly acknowledged or treated during his childhood. Neal had one eye that would turn in toward his nose at times. At the age of 13 Neal underwent eye muscle surgery. His significant struggles with learning and school continued, but his eyes looked straight. Nobody thought that his crossed eye had anything to do with his learning issues, certainly not the eye surgeon. Everyone assumed that the surgery had been successful since his eyes looked normal afterwards. It wasn't given another thought.

It wasn't until 20 years later, just a few months before I would be graduating from optometry school that the truth emerged. We were watching the Super Bowl, which was scheduled to have a 3-D halftime display on television. It was the 1989 Super Bowl halftime show, which was, in Bob Costas's words, "the first ever network broadcast in 3-D." Every 7/11 store was handing out the special 3-D glasses needed to see all the 3-D graphics. I, being a newly minted behavioral optometrist, just happened to have some of my own 3-D glasses that would do the trick. I had two pairs ready for the exciting event - remember, this was in 1989, many years before 3-D movies came back into fashion, so it was going to be something you didn't see very often. My own vision problems made my 3-D experience somewhat muted compared to what it should have been like, but I was seeing 3-D for sure. Some things looked to be closer and some farther away. My brother couldn't figure out what the heck I was talking about. Neal began to describe what he was seeing and it was all just flat.

I decided it would be a good idea to evaluate my brother's vision to see what was going on. Sure enough, the evaluation revealed that even though his eyes appeared straight, Neal was not able to use both eyes in an integrated way.

Long story short, Neal did several months of vision therapy. I was probably more excited than he was when we realized he was finally seeing in 3-D. We continued the vision therapy to ensure that the changes in Neal's visual process would remain intact. It might not have seemed such a big deal at the time, but now Neal is a huge fan of 3-D movies, movies he simply would have been wasting extra money not to see in 3-D without vision therapy.

Nova, My Pride and Joy

I first evaluated Nova, my girlfriend Eva's daughter, shortly after her 5th birthday and shortly after meeting her. Eva had a history of significant nearsightedness in one eye, which is (or should be) a red flag for eye teaming issues. I thought I had noticed Nova's eyes not always looking straight.

Nova's visual evaluation revealed what I had suspected. Her eyes crossed intermittently, sometimes one eye, sometimes the other. Most of the time they were straight. Nova also displayed overall delays in her visual development. In my experience Nova would have been a candidate for eye muscle surgery had she been examined by a surgeon/ophthalmologist. It would not have been surprising for a surgeon to recommend eye muscle surgery even though her eye turn was intermittent and alternating and she could see equally well out of either eye. Her mother might have been told that there was nothing wrong with Nova's eye muscles, but that's how we fix it.

I immediately recommended vision therapy and developmental lenses. I personally oversaw Nova's vision therapy, which consisted of weekly office visits over the course of approximately nine months. I wish I could say that she cooperated in every way, but she did not in fact wear her lenses as much as I would have liked. She did cooperate with the therapy.

Nova and her mother were living in Scotland at the time of her initial evaluation, were only here visiting family, and Nova did not begin vision therapy for several months, once they had permanently relocated to the United States. We became a family at that time and we decided to home school Nova. Eva oversaw the home schooling. Our home schooling program did not have an actual curriculum, but was fairly well-rounded. Nova's home schooling environment included a reasonable amount of socialization, including small groups for math, science and languages as well as two days a week with many other children between the ages of 5 and 13 at a resource center designed to support homeschooling families and stimulate learning and development.

Nova also became involved in sports at age 8; first came soccer and then lacrosse - more on this later. Nova was clearly a very bright child but she was still not reading at age 8. We did not panic, even in the face of constant concern and comments from grandparents and others. We were confident that this would work itself out. Nova decided she wanted to go to school at the age of 10. She wanted to be around the girls she had met through her sports activities and feel more like she was fitting in. Since part of our reasoning for home-schooling was to support independent thinking and behavior, we felt we had an obligation to support Nova's decision, so off to school she went.

Nova immediately thrived in school even though her first experience with it came in the 6th grade - not necessarily the easiest place to jump in. She got excellent grades from that moment forward, and showed significant skill in sports. Nova's soccer coaches did not consider her suitable to play her chosen position - goal keeper, because they said she was too small. What they never found out was that she had incredible ability at the position due to her excellent visual spatial skills, eye/hand coordination, peripheral visual awareness and reaction time. Nova lost interest in soccer because of this and the fact that she was really enjoying playing lacrosse.

Nova was always very active and tom-boyish and bright - and fiercely independent. Vision therapy helped her to make better use of her natural talents. I have no doubt that working on her eye teaming, eye movements and focusing, along with her eye/hand coordination, peripheral vision and reaction time during vision therapy enhanced much of what Nova already had going for her. However, just having natural talent does not guarantee that a person will be able to use those talents fully. Most people are unable to perform up to their potential if the visual process is not operating efficiently. There are plenty of very bright, very talented people out there who are not able to access their assets because their level of visual development is an obstacle and not an advantage. Vision therapy changed that for Nova.

I am immensely proud of Nova, who will be going off to college with both academic and athletic scholarships. She plans on studying law and playing Division 1 lacrosse. Nova is beginning to pack at this very moment.

References

1. Helveston EM. The value of strabismus surgery. Ophthal Surg 1990; 21:311-7.
2. Lipton JR, Willshaw HE. Prospective multicentre study of the accuracy of surgery for horizontal strabismus. Br J Ophthalmol 1995;79:10–11.
3. Kraskin RA. Lens Power in Action. Santa Ana, CA: Optometric Extension Program, Foundation, 2003.
4. Kraskin RA. Personal communication.
5. Barry SR. Fixing My Gaze: A Scientist's Journey into Seeing in Three Dimensions. New Your, NY: Basic Books, 2009.
6. Kitchener G. Personal communication based on the work of Richard Bruenech.
7. Kraskin RA. You Can Improve Your Vision. Santa Ana, CA: Optometric Extension Program, Foundation, 2011. http://oepf.org/product/you-can-improve-your-vision
8. Nelson LB, Calhoun JH, Harley RD, eds, Pediatric Ophthalmology, 3rd ed. Philadelphia: WB Saunders Co., 1991.
9. Wisnicki HJ, Repka MX, Guyton DL . Reoperation rate in adjustable strabismus surgery. J Pediatr Ophthalmol Strabismus 1988;25:112–14.
10. King RA, Calhoun JH, Nelson LB. Reoperations for esotropia. J Pediatr Ophthalmol Strabismus 1987;24:136–40.
11. Kittleman WT, Mazow ML. Reoperations in esotropia surgery. Ann Ophthalmol 1986;18:174-7.
12. Crewther SG, Crewther DP, Mitchell DE, The effects of short-term occlusion therapy on reversal of the anatomical and physiological effects of monocular deprivation in the lateral geniculate nucleus and visual cortex of kittens. Exp Brain Res 1983;51:206-16.
13. Mims JL 3rd, Treff G, Wood RC. Variability of strabismus surgery for acquired esotropia. Arch Ophthalmol 1986;104:1780-2.
14. Kennedy R. McCarthy J. Surgical treatment of esotropia; analysis of case material and results in 315 consecutive cases. Am J Ophthalmol 1959;47:508-19.
15. Maruo T. Nobue K. Iwashige H. Kamiya Y. Long-term results after strabismus surgery. Graefes Arch Clin Exp Ophthalmol 1988;226:414-7.
16. Beneish R. Flanders M. The role of stereopsis and early postoperative alignment in long-term surgical results of intermittent exotropia. Can J Ophthalmol 1994;29:119-24.
17. Teller J. Savir H. Yelin N. Cohen R. Leviav A. Elstin R. Late results of surgery for congenital esotropia. Metab Pediatr Syst Ophthalmol 1988;11:115-8.
18. Greenwald MJ. Amblyopia and Strabismus. Ophthalmol 1987;94:731-5.
19. von Noorden GK. A reassessment of infantile esotropia. Am J Ophthalmol 1988;105:1-10.
20. Spierer A. Binocular function after surgical alignment of infantile esotropia. Metabol Ped Syst Ophthalmol 1988;11:35-6.
21. Pickering JD. Simon JW. Lininger LL. Melsopp KB. Pinto GL. Exaggerated effect of bilateral medial rectus recession in developmentally delayed children. J Pediatr Ophthalmol Strabismus 1994;31:374-7.
22. Capo H, Repka MX, Guyton DL. Hang-back lateral rectus recessions for exotropia. J Pediatr Ophthalmol Strabismus 1989;26:31-4.
23. Makary M. Unaccountable: What Hospitals Won't Tell You and How Transparency Can Revolutionize Health Care. New York: Bloomsbury Press, 2012:52.

Recommended Reading available from Optometric Extension Program Foundation

Fixing My Gaze: A Scientist's Journey Into Seeing in Three Dimensions, by Susan R. Barry

Jillian's Story: How Vision Therapy Changed My Daughter's Life, by Robin and Jillian Benoit

Dear Jillian: Vision Therapy Changed My Life Too, by Robin and Jillian Benoit

The Suddenly Successful Student: A Parents' and Teachers' Guide to Learning & Behavior Problems: How Behavioral Optometry Helps, by Hazel Dawkins, E. Edelman, OD, and C. Forkiotis, OD

Suddenly Successful - How Behavioral Optometry Helps You Overcome Learning, Health And Behavior Problems, by Hazel Dawkins, E. Edelman, OD, and C. Forkiotis, OD

You Can Improve Your Vision, by Robert Kraskin, OD

Lens Power in Action, by Robert Kraskin, OD

Eye Q and the Efficient Learner, by James Kimple

Eyes *OK I'm OK,* by Harold Wiener, OD

Optometric Extension Program Foundation, Inc.
1921 East Carnegie Ave., 3-L
Santa Ana, CA 92705-5811
Online store: www.oepf.org
949 250 8070